A Journey

To Cecile

It was a pleasure
meeting you.
Everything happens for
a reason.
Good Luck on
"your" Journey.

Randy Thompson

A Journey

Serious thoughts about
the search for life
before death

written & illustrated by
Randy Thompson

Canadian Cataloguing in Publication Data

Thompson, Randy, 1957-
 A journey

ISBN 0-9695256-1-3

 1. Thompson, Randy, 1957- 2. Poets, Canadian (English)--20th century--Biography.* I. Title.
PS8589.H5279Z53 1999   C811'.54   C99-910268-0
PR9199.3.T4713Z47 1999

Cover Design by Randy Thompson
Text Layout by Glenys Stuart

Send Correspondence to:
Randy Thompson
P.O. Box 61534
Brookswood Post Office
Langley, B.C.
Canada   V3A 8C8

Listen to Erthtones at:
www.denradio.com/erthtones

Printed and bound in Canada
by Hignell Book Printing.
Printed on acid free recycled paper.

<u>DEDICATION</u>

**This book is dedicated to three special people
who taught me more than they ever realized.
Sadly, their journey ended much too soon.**

My father, Lloyd Fredrick Thompson
October 1929 – May 1979

My brother, Lloyd Fredrick Thompson
July 1954 – February 1992

My son, Thomas Scott William Thompson
December 1985 – May 1988

A Journey

Table of Contents

Foreword

This book has been a long time coming. I'm extremely pleased and proud that it's finally out and in your hands. As you read on, you'll probably agree that this book doesn't easily fit into an exact category. It has poetry in it but it's not really a book of poetry. It talks about my life but it's not exactly an autobiography. It discusses self-improvement but you wouldn't classify it as a self-help book. I guess you could say that it's a poetic self-help autobiography of sorts. Either way, it's unique.

The material in this book was written over a number of years and through different time periods. As you read it, I hope you'll get a sense of where I was at during different times in my life. A lot has changed including this foreword. As I was making some adjustments for the final layout before printing, I read over the old foreword and realized it needed to be updated. Not that there was anything wrong with it per se but my life had changed somewhat. My outlook and philosophy toward respecting nature, others and myself hasn't changed, however what I'm doing in my life has.

Just so you understand where my journey of life has led me, I'll give you a bit of background. My father started a construction company when I was quite young. Even though I chose to go to school to pursue a cooking career, and later on radio broadcasting, I always had a job in construction to go to if

I needed it. Now that may sound like a good thing and the money was all right, but I *hated* the work. I literally *hated* going to work every day. I used to ask myself, "What the hell am I doing here?" The answer usually was "You need to pay your bills so shut up and keep working." I'm happy to say that I no longer work in construction. There isn't anything wrong with construction but, for me, no thank you.

Through a wonderful chain of events, I now find myself working in Film and Television as a background performer and occasionally an actor. I also co-host a radio program on the Internet called Erthtones with a friend of mine, Darryl. Erthtones is intended to be a break from the hectic pace of modern day life. We play earth-beat music and discuss positive, healthy issues and "good news" stories. I'm also involved with a monthly newspaper called "Know News is Good News". The publisher, Nicole, asked me if I would like to contribute a column to the paper. I jumped at the chance and, to my surprise, she dubbed me "The Life Guy". I guess it's just a cross I'll have to bear ☺.

Another aspect of my life that has changed a great deal is my family. To add a little more drama to my life, I'm planning to renew my marriage vows with my wife Patti in Las Vegas this year. We've already said our vows three times together but that's a story in itself! Even though we've had trouble in the past and we actually divorced once, we get along better now than we ever have. My wife and I have also welcomed two new children in to our lives. Harley will be one in March and Shana will be three in March. They join Andrew who will be fifteen in March. Yes, three birthdays within 10 days of each other. A teenager, a toddler and a teether. It's amazing how much energy it takes to change a diaper in the middle of the night once you're past 40! March is an expensive month for us. It ranks right up there with Christmas. There is never a dull moment for us that's for sure. My kids are an inspiration. I'm not saying that they're angels; they're just "real". I'm very thankful for my wonderful wife and my children. I'm humbled by this opportunity to have somewhat of a second chance. I've been given another chance to learn from my mistakes in the past and apply those experiences to enhance my children's futures.

I used to hate my life. Now I love it. I'm thankful that I didn't give up a long time ago. I would have missed so much. I never really know what's going to happen. I never know where my journey is going to take me. Sometimes I have control over it; sometimes things come into my life that I have no control over. That's kind of exciting for me. Obviously there is something to be said for stability and structure but I kind of enjoy that little bit of uncertainty. Up to this point, my journey has been interesting and full of surprises. I hope you enjoy reading about mine as you continue on yours.

ACKNOWLEDGEMENTS

Instead of making a long list of all the people who
have been a part of my journey, I would just like to
acknowledge one special person...
YOU!
(You know who you are!☺)

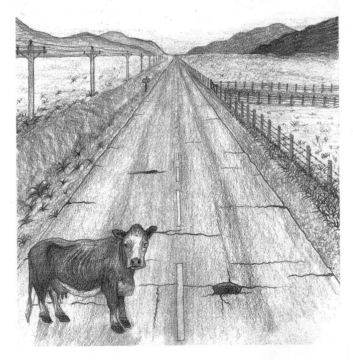

Watch out for cows and potholes on
the journey of life

In the Beginning...

You know, the human race has always confused me. It's ironic that on the one hand human beings are so incredibly intelligent. Look at what we've been able to achieve. We've been able to harness the power of the atom. We've created thousands of machines that can do just about anything we want. We can fly. Well, our machines can. We've gone to the moon and we've sent our machines to the outer reaches of our Solar System. Most of us live in nice warm houses. We can drive to the store and buy just about anything we want. We can eat food produced thousands of miles away, from every corner of the earth. We can instantaneously watch on our televisions whatever is happening on the other side of the planet. We can use an electron microscope to vividly see the most infinitesimal particles. Yes, we're pretty amazing. We've been able to do just about anything we want with things. With objects, with principles, with ideas and theories. We can manipulate and change "things" into whatever we want them to be. We are so intelligent.

But, when it comes to people, to each other, we're really stupid. Okay, wait. I hate that word "stupid." Let's say we're really ignorant. We haven't learned how to treat each other properly. We don't treat each other with respect. Whether it's country to country, social group to social group, religion to religion, race to race or just relating to another person in our life. We more often than not don't treat each other fairly. We're ignorant to the fact that other people have as much right to be here as we do. We often treat each other as garbage. As disposable objects. As "things" that are in our way. We de-humanize people. It's easier that way. We turn them into "things" because we're good with "things". We know how to manipulate and change "things". It's just people that we're terrible with.

So I guess it's a natural response. Good with "things", bad with people. Well, then turn people into "things" and everything will be okay.

But, people aren't "things". They are Human Beings. They have feelings and emotions. They hurt. They cry. They laugh. They think. They love. They hate. They have opinions, and their opinions don't have to agree with yours. That's what has made us so intelligent. We all think differently. We all have our own ideas and we have shared those ideas through the ages. That's how we got to be so good with "things" because we shared our ideas. That's what a library is – a collection of shared ideas.

Imagine if everyone in the world agreed with everything you said and had the same ideas as you. It would be pretty boring, don't you think? We're all individuals. We all have our own ideas and opinions. Just like this book is my opinion. I don't expect you to accept and agree with everything in it. These are my ideas and opinions. I'm merely sharing them with you. If you agree, fine. If you disagree, that's okay too. That just means we're both human.

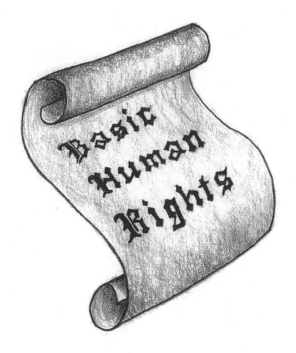

Basic Human Rights

*It doesn't matter how I think
Or what I want to be
I have some basic human rights
Here's what they are to me
I have the right to not go through
Abuse of any kind
I have the right to feelings
And to say what's on my mind
I have the right to not be treated badly by my peers
I have the right to all my pleasures
And to all my fears
I have the right to live my life
The way I want to live
I have the right to take away
I have the right to give
I have the right to worship
In the way that's right for me
I have the right to my beliefs
And the right to be free
I have the right to make mistakes
For that's what humans do
But, when I err, I don't need
To be ridiculed by you
Finally there's one right
Above all else I do expect
No matter if I'm right or wrong
We all deserve respect*

A Journey

This book is about a journey. A journey I've been on my whole life. It's kind of funny because for a long time I didn't even realize I was on one. I thought I was just floating around. Being sent here and put there. Told to sit down and stand up. Do this, do that. I wasn't in control of my own life. I thought everyone else was. I didn't believe I had the right to make decisions for myself without getting approval from someone else. I didn't feel I had the ability to run my own life. I didn't feel much of anything really, except bad. I felt bad about myself. I just basically thought I was pretty much a useless person. Other than feeling bad, I just felt kind of numb. I spent a large part of my life fumbling around, blindly going through the motions of what other people thought I should be doing.

When I look back now, it seems like some strange, surreal movie. I know it's me, playing the role of the "victim" but it's so far removed from how I feel about myself now, it's hard to believe that it actually happened. My self esteem used to be in the toilet, but now I like myself. I'm proud of who I am. I'm glad that I'm here. A far cry from the person who used to drink and do drugs every day, had no self-confidence, didn't like himself, thought he was stupid, felt unworthy of anything, and every once in a while, entertained thoughts of suicide.

It took a long time to get here. I didn't just change overnight. There is a long chain of events that all fit together to get me where I am today. This is my journey but it's not over yet. Not by a long shot. My journey will continue until the day I die and hopefully, beyond that.

It hasn't been easy. Sometimes the easiest thing to do is nothing but if nothing is done, nothing changes. I didn't want to stay the way I was. I wanted to change. I wanted to have a better life. I was tired of feeling bad. I knew I had a problem and I knew I had to do something about it. And so the long process had begun.

I have a tendency to kind of jump around a little bit. So I'm not going to tell you about my journey by starting off by saying "Well, it all began in Hudson Bay, Saskatchewan, where I was born on August 7, 1957 and blah, blah, blah..." That would be kind of boring. So I'll skip a whole pile of stuff and bounce from this to that and go from here to there and I promise, that in the end, it will all make sense. Well, at least I hope it will.

So let's take a jump to a time which explains how I started this whole "book" idea. Back in 1990, I had been going to a support group, A.C.O.A. (Adult Children of Alcoholics). I started writing poems and sharing them at meetings. The response I got really amazed me. People said they could relate to my poems and started asking for copies of them. I began photocopying what I had and, after a while, I thought, "Why don't I just write a book?" Eventually, that's what I did. I originally published a book of my poetry titled "Serious Thoughts About the Search for Life Before Death. Words of a Recovering Human Being" (1990). Most of the poems in that book are also in this one, along with many new ones.

The first poem in that book was called "Dad". I put it first because a lot of people said it sounded just like their dad. It seems as though many people still have unresolved issues with their parents, especially their fathers. They seem to have been deeply affected by the way they were raised. I used to use the word dysfunctional a lot but I try to stay away from it now. It has become really overused and when it comes right down to it, we're all pretty much dysfunctional. I started looking at it more in terms of an unbalanced, unsafe, emotionally unhealthy family environment. Being raised like this, coupled with one or more forms of abusive treatment, will have a negative effect on just about anybody.

"Mankind" has done a great disservice to himself. He has heaped a huge burden on his own shoulders. For generations, men and boys have been told "Don't show your emotions. Keep it all inside. Don't be a wimp. Straighten up there. Don't show them your weak side." It has really screwed us males up. Things are changing a bit now, but for ages men have been afraid to be vulnerable. They've been afraid to be wrong. They've been afraid of making mistakes for fear of looking weak. Essentially being human. Let's face it, we ARE vulnerable. We CAN be wrong. We DO make mistakes and sometimes we ARE weak. We DON'T know all the answers although sometime we like to THINK we do. It's like the jokes about men not wanting to ask for directions and REAL men don't need instructions. Men don't want to look like they don't know something. That's why those jokes are funny because they're true.

Dad

I wish you were still here today
There's lots of things I'd like to say

Like gosh-darn shucks... I love you Dad
Your absence truly makes me sad

I never really got to see
The real you... He was kept from me

Your image was to just be strong
Don't cry and don't admit you're wrong

Don't show your feelings, most of all
For that is weak... Be tough... Stand tall

But I know that deep down inside
There was a child you used to hide

Sometimes he'd come out... want to play
But all too soon be locked away

Dad, I know that you've been hurt
I know you've been dragged through the dirt

You did the best that you could do
You passed on what was done to you

But I wish you were here today
So you and I could go and play

A Journey

My father passed away from a heart attack in 1979. I was 21 at the time. Unfortunately, I never got the chance to know my father as a person. He was always in the stern role of "Father". As his son, I never really felt I measured up to his expectations. I felt like I was a disappointment to him. He would never tell me that he loved me. He wouldn't say he was proud of me. If I did something well, he would ignore it. If I did something wrong, he would be on my ass in a second. There was total lack of positive reinforcement and heavy negative reinforcement. After a while I thought, "Can't I do anything right?" I started to approach everything from the angle of "What's wrong with it" instead of "What's right with it". I began to focus on the negative instead of on the positive.

Now, I don't want to paint my father as the "Bad Guy". He was a very intelligent, talented, articulate, hard working man. But he was carrying all that "Man Stuff". He didn't want us to see his weak side. I know now that he loved me very much. I just didn't know it then. I know that he was very proud of me. He had a hard time letting out his feelings. He could tell you what he thought, but he had trouble telling you what he felt.

My father owned his own successful construction company. I chose to become a chef. We were going to start a restaurant together. He wanted to call it "Randy's". It's too bad. It could have been great, but then again, who knows? Having my father as a business partner might not have been such a good idea.

I understand now what his motivations were.

Sometimes his methods were a bit counter-productive, but he just wanted me to grow up to be the best person I could be.

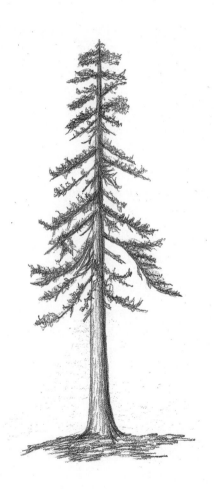

New Beginning*

The Human mind's a wonderful recorder
It stores everything you see and do
But sometimes painful memories get blocked out
Some memories of abuse just don't get through

You end up thinking "What's the matter with me?"
These thoughts I have are awfully bizarre
I have to keep these thoughts of mine a secret
I can't let anyone know what they are

For if they see inside me, they won't like me
I'm full of all this ickyness inside
I wish I didn't have to make a living
For all I want to do is run and hide

My needs don't really seem very important
What other people want always comes first
I keep myself extended into their needs
Ignore my needs and treat myself the worst

I let these people walk all over my face
I find it really hard to just say... NO
I'd like to just relax and take it easy
But they say – Can You? and Zip... off I go

I really wish I was a better person
Instead of one who always gets the blame
I feel the guilt of things of which I'm guiltless
People call me stupid and fill me with shame

I wish my mind could slow down for a minute
It's racing here and then it's racing there
Reliving and rehashing all my mistakes
And the torment in my life I've had to bear

It's not my fault, I really didn't mean it
I didn't want to hurt the ones I did
You people, you all see me as an adult
But inside I'm just a frightened little kid

It seems that when I love someone, I hurt them
I don't mean to, it just seems to work that way
I'll get involved with someone that attracts me
Very quickly I'll just want to pull away

For in the past, my feelings have been stepped on
In relationships I always seem to lose
I always find exactly the same person
In every new relationship I choose

I like to spend a lot of time by myself
I often want to have no one around
For if I'm all alone, no one can hurt me
And alone has been the safest place I've found

But all alone, there is no one to talk to
To laugh with, or to cry with, or to share
It's true there is no one to shame or hurt me
But there's also no one there to show they care

A Journey

I've built this wall, this fortress, all around me
To protect me from the painful, harsh, cruel world
But in defense, my fortress has been transformed
And before me, my own prison has unfurled

I'm trapped inside myself, and I just want out
I want to end this madness that's my life
I have a last resort but I don't like it
I've never liked the combo-wrists and knife

But if I kill myself I'll just be quitting
And I'll never get to be a big success
I'll never feel a kiss, a hug, a handshake
And I'll never feel another warm caress

So maybe suicide is not the answer
It's too messy and too final, anyway
Before I go I think I'll try that group thing
What's their name again? Oh ya! A.C.O.A.

* One of my first poems, written early in my recovery.

Obviously I had a pretty low self-esteem. Most of my life I felt I didn't fit in, I didn't belong. In elementary school, I didn't have many friends. I was very quiet and spent a lot of time by myself. A large part of my alienation came from my size. I was always the biggest person in my class. I'm 6' 4" now. At the age of 12 I was 150 pounds. Size can automatically be intimidating. People usually equate big people with small brains (if you're big, you must be stupid). My peers would often ridicule me and call me stupid. I guess it made them feel better about themselves. The trouble was, I already felt bad about myself because of some abuse issues and the ridicule just reinforced my low self-esteem. If people tell you you are stupid for long enough you take that on as your identity. You become what people tell you you are. After a while, you just give up trying because you begin to believe what they tell you. "Why bother, because I'm stupid." Then, when they stop calling you down, you keep doing it to yourself. If I made a mistake I would say to myself "What's the matter with me? How could I be so stupid?" I would reinforce my own negative self-image. Sometimes it amazes me how we treat each other and ourselves.

Shaming Words

I overheard a woman say
"You're ROTTEN" to her child one day
I thought, 'How sad, that's really wild.
To talk that way to your own child.'
I will not play that hurtful game
Of passing on your guilt and shame
I show my son Love and Respect
His needs I try not to neglect
I say "I Love You" every day
The shaming words I will not say
For words can be a vicious thing
I've felt the pain that they can bring

My father helped keep the "stupid" image going by always pointing out my mistakes. Something he would always say was "Make sure your brain is engaged before your mouth is in gear". My brother didn't help a lot either. Lloyd was the aggressive, hyper, abusive older brother. He was three years older than me. We fought all the time. I almost always lost. Not necessarily physically, but I lost mentally and emotionally. Lloyd, and to some extent my Dad, could manufacture anger at will and bring it up when they needed it. No matter how angry I got, they could just go to the next level of anger and always be angrier than I was. I would just fold up and crawl away under the onslaught.

Anger

There's an issue I must address
About the anger I don't express

I keep my feelings trapped inside
It's almost like I've cheated, lied

I haven't let my true self shine
A bigger anger suppresses mine

I feel – 'Why bother, there is no hope'
For faced with anger, it's hard to cope

I'll push mine down, won't let it show
But now frustration starts to grow

My anger builds and eats away
It clouds my thoughts from day to day

Can't clear my head, can't get things done
Just want to live, to have some fun

But there it is, that great big wall
It looks so tough, it seems so tall

But, all I have to do is "be"
To let out what's inside of me

To say exactly how I feel
To show myself my anger's real

I can't ignore my inner self
I've spent too long upon the shelf

I'm coming down to live my life
I've been so full of stress and strife

It's time to let my feelings flow
And finally, I can start to grow

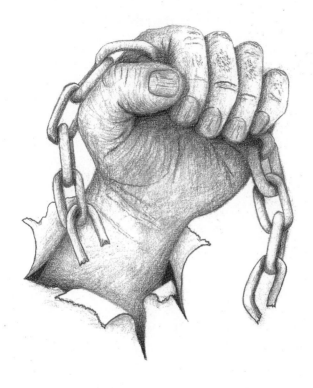

Breaking the bonds of self-imprisonment

My state of mind got pretty low at times. It just seemed like there was no way out. All this crap just kept piling up and I didn't know how to cope with it. I used to beat myself up mentally all the time about mistakes I was making. I would dwell on things for ages. I would carry something around in my mind and I wouldn't forgive myself. The only time I would forget about it was when I had some new "bigger" mistake to dwell on. After a while I couldn't take it anymore. I started thinking about the "S" word. Suicide. The only thing that stopped me was I knew if I killed myself it would have devastated my mother. So I didn't.

Thanks Mom.

Recovery Begins...

I'm Glad I Never Killed Myself

I'm glad I never killed myself
The way I almost did
Sometimes the pain just seemed too much
Come on! I'm just a kid
Why do these people want to hurt?
They like to see me crawl
I never did a thing to them
It's not my fault, at all
I just can't take it anymore
I have to find an out
I'll toast myself. Yeah! Suicide
And then THEY'LL cry and shout
I'll show them that it's all their fault
And boy, will they be sorry
I just might even make the NEWS
I'll be a front page story...

But now I'm glad I'm here today
To store these words for you
I'm glad I never killed myself
I'm glad I stuck it through
For through my pain I've seen the light
My life was not a waste
Today my life is wonderful
I didn't act in haste
No matter how depressed you get
It isn't worth your life
Sometimes there's pain, sometimes there's joy

Sometimes there's stress and strife
I'm glad I never killed myself
I'm glad I'm here today
I'm glad that I went through that pain
And through it is the only way

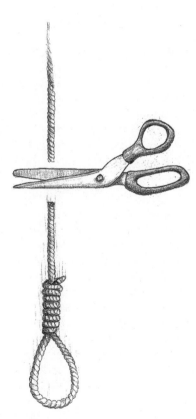

Well, if I couldn't kill myself I just did the next best thing. I numbed myself out. Alcohol and Drugs. That became my main priority. First time I ever got drunk I was 12. All through my teen years every weekend I spent drinking and smoking. Not tobacco – marijuana was my drug of choice. I never did heroin and I never used a needle, although I tried just about everything else. Cocaine, LSD, MDA, Mescaline, Peyote buttons, Opium, Uppers, Downers. I even used to grow my own Magic Mushrooms. I experimented but I stayed pretty much a pothead and a drinker.

I can't begin to count the number of times I should have been killed. I fell asleep at the wheel, twice, drunk of course, and wrecked two cars. Not that I'm proud of it but, for the record, I've estimated that I must have driven legally impaired close to 2000 times. I thank God that luckily I didn't hurt anyone. I just ran into inanimate objects. I drank every day – I drove every day.

Drinking just became a way of life. It's what I did. I used to say, "I don't drink before noon." As time went by I'd crack a beer for breakfast and say, "Well, it must be noon somewhere." Alcohol became a friend, a companion. It was always there to comfort me, to give me confidence. It was almost like having a relationship with someone. Alcohol became my Significant Other. I went everywhere with her. She was always with me. I knew where all the liquor stores were. I knew when all the bars opened. I used to drink vodka secretly, beer openly.

For a long period of time I always kept a bottle of vodka in my truck and mixed it with pop. That way I could drink and drive and no one really noticed.

Now, my drinking wasn't always that bad. It progressed slowly through my teens. Then, when I became "legal" it was a regular thing to go to the bar after work to socialize with the guys. It was a "social" thing. That's what I wanted to believe anyway. Gradually it became what I did every day. I used to think about quitting and I would wonder, "Is there life after NOT drinking?" Would I be able to handle going through life without alcohol? Would life be really boring without it? But it got to the point where it became obvious I couldn't keep going like this. I had to do something.

I decided to go for Drug and Alcohol counselling in 1986. At my second session, my counsellor asked me why I like drinking. I had to really think about it. I told him I like that feeling I get when I have my first drink. It just feels nice. So he said, "Well, then just have one drink and stop. See how that goes." So that's what I did.

I was working at CHWK in Chilliwack as a radio announcer doing the late shift. I got off work at midnight, went to a local nightclub and had one drink. I had a double vodka soda. To me, that was one drink. I played pool. I wanted another drink. The evening was over. I wanted another one. I went home. I really wanted another one. I did the same thing the next night and it was even worse. I was going nuts. I WANTED ANOTHER DRINK. Sitting there in that tiny apartment I realized that I can't control this. I can't

A Journey

have just one and be comfortable. One is not enough. And if I have more than one, I know what will happen.

The next night I had planned to drive to Surrey after work. As I was driving down the highway, my water pump exploded right at the entrance of the only rest stop on that entire stretch of road. I coasted in and parked. It was about 2 a.m. An older gentleman by the name of Harvey pulled in and offered me a ride to Surrey. As he drove, we had an in-depth conversation about our lives. It was amazing. It was as if we had lived the same life. He also had problems with alcohol and had quit drinking seven years earlier. As long as I live, I'll never forget what he said to me. His words were: "You're lucky to be this young and to be able to see your problem because I wasted a lot of years." And WHAM!!!!! It was just like someone turned on the light. It was like I could see for the very first time.

We got to where he was dropping me off and I didn't want to get out of the car. We sat there and talked for another hour. That was July 6, 1986. I've never had a drink since and I've never really wanted one. I don't mean to make it seem like quitting drinking is easy. I know it's not easy for a lot of people. It's a lifelong struggle. My heart and admiration goes out to anyone who is battling addiction and wants to improve themselves. I just wanted to be a better person. I was tired of what I was doing to myself. I knew that if I was going to quit, I was just going to have to QUIT. I couldn't have one or two drinks and be comfortable so I just wouldn't have any. I knew what would happen if I did, so I just said, "NO, I HAVE TO STOP THIS". I changed the way I saw the whole thing. I gained a totally different perspective that night. I realized later one of the reasons it was easier for me was because I did a couple of "steps" without even knowing anything about the Twelve Step Program.

In the Twelve Step Program, Step 1 is you admit that you are powerless over Alcoholism and/or the dysfunction of your family, that your life had become unmanageable. I did that when I realized I couldn't control my drinking. Then, I kind of did Step 5 when I met Harvey. Step 5 being admitting to God, to myself and to another Human Being the exact nature of my wrongs.

Now, I'm not going to say that on July 6, 1986, I stopped all addictive, destructive behaviour. About six months after that, I slowly started smoking pot again and held on to that for a couple of years. I guess I still needed to hold onto something. I quit smoking pot on March 6, 1989.

I Used To Smoke Pot

*I used to smoke pot
I used to drink booze
No matter what I tried
I always would lose*

*I kept myself "numbed" out
From feeling the pain
It seemed life was worthless
There was nothing to gain*

*I'll just sit here stoned
And let life go by
I'm going to lose anyway
So why bother to try*

*I'll stay in my corner
Back up to the wall
Why stand up and walk?
When through life I can crawl*

*May not be fulfilling
It's all that I've got
I'll hold onto this crutch
For stable, I'm not*

*It must be someone's fault
It sure can't be mine
I'll numb myself out
With this joint and this wine...*

But now I can see
How I erred, I was wrong
For life is too short
Yes it's not very long

Think positive
That is the best train of thought
I'm glad I can say that...
I USED TO smoke pot

A Journey

Now I don't believe that my water pump just happened to explode at the only rest stop on the highway. And I don't believe that Harvey just happened to drive in to the rest stop at 2 a.m. and offer me a ride. Or we just happened to have the most stimulating conversation of my entire life. There was a long chain of events that put that whole thing together. I do not believe it was a random chain of events. It wasn't coincidence. I believe it was meant to happen for whatever reason. I don't believe in fate as in your whole life is planned out ahead of time. I believe there is a higher power watching over us all. I believe God, Great Spirit, Jesus, Mohammed, Allah, Buddha, Krishna or whatever you want to call it, is nudging things here, putting things there and placing things in an order that has a purpose. I do not believe that events are random.

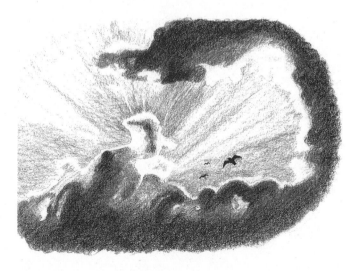

Events

There is an order to the way
Events unfold from day to day
Things happen and you don't *know* why
But then it's clear as time goes by
Events all seem to have their place
So just slow down...Life's not a race
For what is TRULY meant to be
Will soon become reality

Even though I no longer drink nor do drugs, I am not an avid non-drinker. If someone wants to have a couple of drinks that's okay with me. There are lots of people who don't have a problem with it. Just because you drink doesn't mean you're an alcoholic. On the other hand, I don't like to see people who do have a problem with alcohol or drugs continue to abuse them. There are many ways that people can display alcoholism. They may binge drink as in drink only on the weekends. They may drink every day. They may drink openly or secretly. They could drink beer or wine or whatever. They may feel they "need" alcohol to maintain their composure. That's what I did for a long time. I was a maintenance drinker. I maintained a level of alcohol in my system so I could continue functioning. I felt I needed it. Alcoholism can manifest itself in many ways.

My drug and alcohol counsellor gave me a general guideline for alcoholism. If, when you drink, it affects you in an adverse way as in it changes your behaviour and personality, there is probably reason to be concerned. Now, of course if someone goes and gets drunk and does something silly, that's not necessarily what I mean, but if there is a consistent shift in behaviour when someone's drinking there could be a problem.

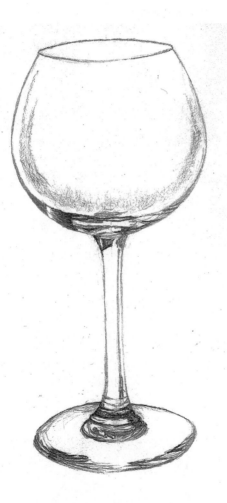

Waste

There's something that I see today
Most everywhere I turn
There's people wasting everything
It seems they never learn

They're wasting paper and tin cans
They're wasting plastic too
They're wasting glass and energy
They waste things old and new

Of all the things that people waste
The worst one that I find
Are people who are stuck on drugs
They're wasting their own mind

Now listen, I'm no angel
And I don't profess to be
I've done a lot of drugs myself
Today though, I'm drug-free

It took me oh so many years
But finally I have faced
That a human mind is simply
Just an awful thing to waste

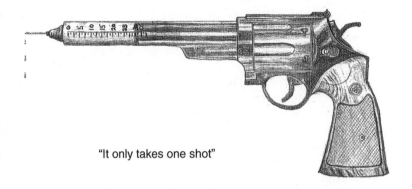

"It only takes one shot"

It was kind of strange after I quit drinking and doing drugs. I started living my life without worrying about running out of pot or thinking about going to the bar. No hangovers. I started getting in touch with feelings I had pushed down for a long time. I started feeling better about myself. I started feeling worse about myself. I started feeling.

For most of my life I had been wearing emotional blinders. Not only had I been protecting myself from the outside world, I had also been protecting myself from myself. I had been afraid to allow myself to feel the world around me. I had been afraid of being hurt again. The easiest way to not be hurt by feelings is to not feel anything at all. That's why I had relied so heavily on alcohol and drugs. It was a way of numbing out my feelings and keeping reality at bay. Now that I no longer had the "protection" of any intoxicants and I was moving towards improving myself, I had no choice but to face the feelings.

Feeling

I cried today and it was good
I felt I was alive
I'm feeling more as time goes by
In fact, my feelings thrive

I've spent the past all numb inside
I couldn't feel a thing
I thought I knew what feelings were
But now the truth doth ring

I see now that I've fooled myself
By believing what was wrong
I felt that I was "bad" and "weak"
But now I know I'm STRONG

It's nice to feel what's all around
The good stuff and the bad
For now instead of being "numb"
I'm "happy" and I'm "sad"

There's ups in life and then there's downs
There's tears and laughter too
And "FEELING" beats "NUMB" any day
And "FEELING" is what I'll do

Now, just because I quit alcohol and drugs it didn't mean my life was great. There were still all the reasons I numbed myself out in the first place. I didn't even understand them. I just didn't feel good about myself.

Someone observing my people-pleasing behaviour one day asked me if my parents drank. I said, "yes, they both do." She promptly replied, "Well, then you're an Adult Child of an Alcoholic." She briefly explained the Adult Child Phenomenon and what the support group A.C.O.A. was about. I initially rejected the idea but found it interesting. I filed it in the back of my mind.

Shortly after that, I got a job at Cariboo Radio in Quesnel as a radio announcer. One night I was read-ing a Community Service Announcement on the air that went something like this: "Quesnel A.C.O.A. Support Group meets Monday nights in the Quesnel Library." I thought, "Wow...divine intervention. It's being sent to me." So, of course, I went. When I even-tually moved back to Richmond, I hooked up with the Richmond A.C.O.A group. No one, including me, can speak for all A.C.O.A. groups as a whole, but in my experience, it was a place I could go to, listen to other people's experience and express myself in a safe, non-judgmental environment. A.C.O.A. is a support group based on the Twelve Steps of Alcohol-ics Anonymous. What I gained most from A.C.O.A. was the understanding that I wasn't alone. When I listened to people speak about themselves, I heard my own life unfolding. I always thought it was just me. I thought I was the only one going through this stuff. I thought I was the only one that felt this way. I started to feel connected. I started to feel a healing process begin. I wasn't alone anymore.

I started to really take an honest look at myself. I never wanted to do that before. It was too painful. It was easier to just deny there was a problem in the first place. They say denial is just like an onion – you start peeling it down one layer at a time. As you start to deal with one layer, you expose another one deeper down. Recovery is like that onion. You keep peeling down through your layers and begin to uncover stuff you might not even have known existed.

For me, it was exciting and scary at the same time. Even though it was uncomfortable talking about, remembering, and to some extent re-living some painful periods in my life, it felt as though I was beginning to gain my freedom. I didn't feel so weighed down anymore. I could see that there was hope after all.

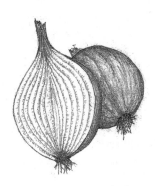

To Share

To share means help
To share means love
To share means ease the pain
To share means giving of yourself
To share means much to gain
To share means you extend your hand
To someone who's in need
To share means acting out of love
And never hate or greed
To share is an unselfish act
To share means "I am here
To help you through this painful time"
And maybe share a tear
Yes, when you share of what you have
People will share with you
I've learned to share my joy and pain
I will my whole life through

The Best Trip

There's many things that I have seen
There's lots of places I have been

Yes, I have travelled far and wide
But, there's one trip I hadn't tried

I hadn't searched inside my soul
Conceal myself, that was my goal

"Don't look at who you really are"
"Forget it, just go to the bar"

"A couple of beers, it goes away"
"Tomorrow is another day"

But days all melted into one
I wasn't having any fun

I don't drink now, it's been four years
And in that time I've shed some tears

I've searched my soul, I've looked inside
I tell the truth, now I don't hide

I've found the truth, I've seen the light
Now I am on a joyous flight

Of all the places I could be
The best trip is recovery

The concept of being an Adult Child is as a child, your needs weren't properly met. Whether it be physically, emotionally, spiritually or mentally, you weren't nurtured in a healthy environment. You don't have to come from an alcoholic family to become, (here goes that word), dysfunctional. It could be from abuse (sexual, physical, emotional, mental, ritual), neglect, abandonment or whatever leaves you feeling unsafe, unloved or unwanted. It can have a serious effect on your emotional stability. As a result, when that emotionally unstable child grows up, they become an emotionally unstable adult. There's still that little child inside who feels afraid, unsafe and unloved. But most of all, unworthy. The little child inside internalizes everything and blames themselves. "It's all my fault".

Over the years, I've heard the phrase "Inner Child" used a lot. When something new begins to become main stream, it can be irritating to some people. I've heard jokes made about the "Inner Child" like "What your Inner Child needs is a good spanking." You can call it what you want but we really don't have any other words that describe what I think the "Inner Child" is. To me it is your emotional center. It's the person who talks to you in your head. It's the part of you that has fun if you allow yourself to play. It's the part that loves roller coasters or hates them. It's the part of you that feels the fear. A surprise birthday or a power outage on a stormy night would certainly evoke different emotional responses. I believe it's the "Inner Child" that reacts emotionally to those situations. Who your "Inner Child" is and how they react depends on your physical and emotional experiences. Some people deny themselves the fun part of life and always act very "Adult"-like. Other people act very childlike all the time. I believe that there is a healthier balance somewhere in the middle. As an adult I do have to act responsibly and adult-like some of the time. There are other times that I need to just play and have fun.

"You Gotta Listen To Your Inner Child"

(I wrote this as a song)

There is a person inside of you
Who's just a kid, nothin' you can do
Has been there forever, your whole life through

I'm talking about your Inner Child
Oh yes, I said I'm talkin' about your Inner Child

Your child feels happy
Your child feels sad
Your child is joyous
Your child gets mad
Sometime it's furious
Sometimes glad

Oh, talkin' about your Inner Child
Oh ya, I'm talkin' about your Inner Child

Don't lock away your Inner Child
You gotta listen to your Inner Child

Your child remembers all the pain you've been through
Your child also remembers the fun things too
But joy and fun might be foreign things to you

Just listen to your Inner Child
Oh ya, you gotta listen to your Inner Child

Well, sometimes angry
And sometimes mild
Sometimes meek

A Journey

And then sometimes wild
Knows all the secrets that you keep filed

Said talkin' about your Inner Child
Oh yes, you gotta listen to your Inner Child

When memories are painful, then sometimes you hide
Your true inner self, it's a matter of pride
Can't let people see the real you inside

There's one person in the world that you just can't fool
Don't lie to your child, that can be so cruel
Just dwell in the truth, it's a golden rule

Be truthful with your Inner Child
Ya gotta listen to your Inner Child
Start talkin' to your Inner Child
Go golfin' with your Inner Child
Have pizza with your Inner Child
Play checkers with your Inner Child
Have some fun with your Inner Child
Try laughin' with your Inner Child
And cryin' with your Inner Child
But don't forget about your Inner Child

Not everyone reacts to the same situation the same way. We all have different personalities. Everyone has their own history with their own unique combination of events and experiences. I believe most of us have suffered some kind of abuse at one time or another in our lives most probably as a child. Abuse comes in many forms and varies widely in severity. It seems fairly clear to me that abuse can have a negative effect on how people see themselves and the world around them. Not all self-image and self-esteem problems stem from abuse but it seems a good proportion do. It's difficult for some people to let go of the past and move forward in a healthy way after being mistreated by people they trusted. When the issue of abuse comes up, I've heard people say things like, "All that stuff was in the past"; "Stop thinking about it"; "Get on with your life"; and "Just forget about it".

Well, that may be easy to say but it's not always so easy to do. When you're talking about your self-image, it's pretty hard to just change the way you see yourself. It's been your whole life up to that point. It's all you've ever known. It's who you are. All the events in your life have contributed to who you are today. It's not easy to just "forget about it". I always said it's like dragging around a huge ball and chain. You don't see it, you're not looking at it, but as you move through your life, it's affecting everything you do. You need to turn around, look at it, face it, and deal with it. Make some healthy choices.

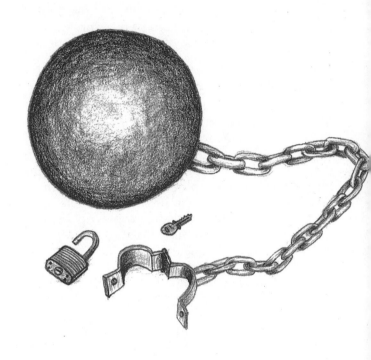

You have the key

Choices

A choice is something that 'I' make
I see now that it's mine

I have the right to make my own
To let my Choices shine

If I choose stuff that's bad for me
Then I'll be hurt again

But I can choose the healthy things
Things that won't cause me pain

To take responsibility
And do what's best for me

I find is new, and hard to do
But I want to be free

I'm going to give myself the best
The things that I deserve

Why do things that are bad for me?
What purpose would that serve?

A choice is something that 'I' make
No one can pull my strings

I'm going to choose what's best for me
I choose the healthy things

I began to realize I couldn't go back and change the past. I couldn't change the fact that I had made some big mistakes in my life. Sometimes it's hard to look back through the events in your life and take responsibility for your actions. It's often easier to blame something or someone else or some extenuating circumstances. It's easier to minimize your involvement, downplay your own part in it or deny you even had anything to do with it. The hard part is to openly say, "I screwed up. I made a mistake. I'm sorry." It slowly dawned on me that I WAS involved. I DID do it. This was MY history. I own it. It's my past (problem) and no one else's. I have to take responsibility for it whatever it may be. I have to be honest with myself and realize I can't change the past. I CAN change the way I see things. I can admit and own my actions and words.

Something I don't want to do is repeat my mistakes from the past. By being honest with myself, I can learn from those mistakes. Instead of constantly berating myself for making the same mistakes over and over, I could use my mistakes as lessons in life like they were meant to be. I needed to start forgiving myself for the errors I was making and learn to accept myself. Something that helped me in that area was a few weekend retreats that I went on up the Chilliwack River. These retreats were intense support group weekends. We did different exercises covering different issues. One of those exercises was very simple yet very powerful. We all sat around the fire pit and introduced ourselves by saying, "Hi. I'm

Randy and I love and accept myself." Now that may
sound easy but some people couldn't even say the
words. They didn't accept themselves and they didn't
love themselves. It was a bit of a breakthrough for
me because even though I could say the words, I
knew I didn't believe them. It forced me to look at
the fact that I really didn't love and accept myself.
It's difficult to accept yourself after disliking who you
are for so long.

It took a while but I started giving myself the
benefit of the doubt. Slowly I stopped beating myself
up about the past. I started moving forward and
began feeling a lot better about myself. I realized
that there was hope. I was on the right path. I felt
like I was turning into the person that I was supposed to be. It felt good. I wasn't ashamed of who I
was anymore. I hadn't changed my past. I had just
changed the way I looked at it. I had changed the
way I felt about myself.

Myself –Today

*I've learned too much, I won't go back to
where I used to be.
I lived a life of pain, addiction, hurt and
misery.
I had no self-esteem and no self-worth, no
self-respect.
I practiced self-abuse and self-destruction,
self-neglect.
I've come so far, I like myself. Quite differ-
ent from the past.
Back then everything else came first and
my needs always last.
I also hurt the ones I loved. In that there
is no glory.
I caused a lot of pain myself, for that I'm
truly sorry.
And I know that I can't go back and
change those things.
Not one.
They're now a part of History. They can-
not be undone.
I can't go back, I won't go back and live
my life that way.
I know that there's one thing that I "can"
change:
"Myself – Today".*

I'm Proud

*Most of my life, I didn't try
To do what's best. I now know why
I didn't feel that I had worth
Sometimes regretted my own birth
But, now I'm proud of what I do
I'm proud of where I'm going to
I now do what is best for me
I'm proud I'm in recovery*

A Journey

For most of my life, I was always concerned about what everyone else thought. "I better not do that or say this. Someone else might not like it. What if they didn't like me? What if they come right out and say something bad about me? I don't think I could handle the rejection." I was always cautious about what I said and did in the hopes that I would be accepted. In the hope that I would fit in. Now I realize that what other people think and say about me isn't important. It's what I think and say about myself that matters.

An event that vividly showed me that it didn't matter anymore what other people thought took place in a playground with my son who was only six at the time. He was climbing on the monkey bars and I was swinging on a swing. I've always enjoyed that kind of play but never allowed myself to do it because someone else might think I was too big for it. Well, sure enough, a car drove by and from the passenger seat window a rather large man yelled out, "Don't you think you're a little big for that?" Without even thinking about it, I yelled back at the top of my lungs, "No!" I just started laughing. It was such an exhilarating feeling. I was free! It didn't matter anymore. Why should I care what he thinks? It's a moment I'll always cherish. At that instant I realized that everything was going to be all right. All I had to do was just be ME.

Now And Then

I take a look. I breathe a sigh.
I notice how the time's gone by.
I'm not the person that I was.
I know I'm not; I'm not because
My thoughts have changed so radically
I feel the peace and joy in me.
Back then I just wanted to hide
But now my heart is full of pride.
I love the person I've become –
I now know where I'm coming from.
Yes, God has seen the good in me.
I thank him for recovery.

A Journey

Growing up, I usually tried to be funny. Sometimes I acted like the class clown so I could make people laugh. If I made people laugh at what I was saying or doing, they wouldn't be laughing at me as a person. By drawing attention to myself I drew attention away from me. I had been keeping reality at bay by turning everything into a joke.

Once I started taking a real look at myself, I realized I had been using humour as a defense. I was always trying to "entertain". I had trouble carrying on a serious conversation. I would make jokes constantly. I was playing the comedian. My mind was always looking for the pun or the punchline. After making a joke once when my wife was trying to be serious, she yelled with frustration, "Can't you be serious about anything?" At that moment I realized there was a problem. You can be TOO funny. Not everything is a joke. So I decided to stop being funny altogether. I became very serious. I didn't want to use humour as a way of hiding. For a long time, I didn't make jokes about anything. After a while I began to see that it wasn't the humour that was inappropriate, it was just the way I had been using it that was inappropriate. I was way out of balance.

I love humour. I still love to make people laugh. Now I make jokes and humorous comments when it's more appropriate but I can also be very serious. I realized there has to be a balance.

Balance

*You know, too much of anything just isn't
good for you.*
*You have to find the balance in most every-
thing you do.*
*You might enjoy a little wine; that's perfectly
alright.*
*But don't go to the bar and get polluted
every night.*
*You might like to party and spend all your
time with friends*
But your responsibility to family never ends.
*We need to eat. It's how we live. We need
food, one and all.*
*But diets high in fat will jack up your
cholesterol.*
*We need to work so we get paid and buy the
things we lack,*
*But too much work can stress you out – give
you a heart attack.*
*There's lots of things that we abuse. There's
things we do too much*
*Like sex and drugs and work and play. They
can become a crutch.*
*All things in moderation is the order of
the day.*
*We have to find the balance between work
and home and play.*
*There needs to be some give and take – not
too much nor too little–*

*We need to find the balance point. It's some-
where in the middle.
So try to find the balance in all the things
you do.
They say, "too much of anything just isn't
good for you."*

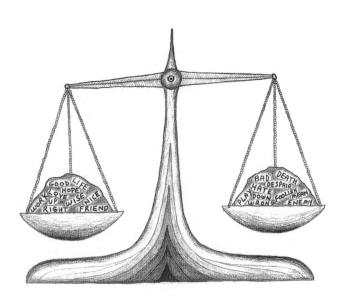

I used to waste a lot of time. I didn't really use my time wisely. I used to make the joke "I bought a book on Effective Time Management but I just can't find the time to read it." When you're practicing addiction, most of your time is used looking for the money, looking for the stuff, getting the stuff, using the stuff, feeling the buzz, coming down and then starting the cycle all over again. It's all about "me". Nothing else matters. Who cares about anything else?

It was nice to look around and begin to enjoy life. To focus on the good things, the positive things. To see the world with a clear, unclouded head. I began to see there was lots of work that had to be done on myself, in my life, with my family, in my community, in this country and in the world. I couldn't afford to waste too much time. Once time has gone by, you can never get it back.

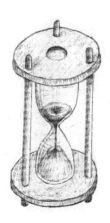

Today

Don't put off until tomorrow
What you can do today
I'm sure you've heard those words before
An overworked cliché
But there's a lot of wisdom that's
Contained within that phrase
The essence of it is to be
Productive with your days
To look at the reality of
Life for you and me
You'll see that yesterday is gone
Tomorrow's yet to be
So live life one day at a time
And learn along the way
Remember yesterday is gone
So do your best today

Something that was becoming very clear to me was how this abuse, low self-esteem, dysfunctional cycle keeps moving down through families – through generations. It gets passed down from one level to the next and from one person to the other. It's like unloading your garbage onto the next one in line because your load is too heavy. It's called scapegoating. Attacking a person or group in order to feel cleansed of feelings of sadness, helplessness, inadequacies and anxieties. Unfortunately, it is somewhat true that you always hurt the ones you love. Everyone else is too far away, too distant but your family members are right there within arm's reach. Some people tend to vent their frustrations at the ones who are closest to them. It certainly isn't fair but it somehow feels "safer" to let go around family members because they've always been there and have always accepted it.

I decided I didn't want to be just a link in that familial chain. I wanted to break the cycle of pain, shame and abuse. I didn't want to pass anything down to my son that was unhealthy. Children learn by example. I couldn't just tell him how to behave and then show him something different. You know, the old, "Don't do what I do, do as I say" adage. I realized I had to be a good model for him. I had to set a good example.

Example

It hurts me to see I've affected my son
I've passed on dysfunction to my little one

I've given him traits that are inside of me
But it's not my fault because I didn't see

I just acted out from the things in my past
Things happen so quickly and time moves so fast

But now I do see I can change what I've done
Life can be much better for my little son

But things won't improve if I try to fix him
It'll take much hard work, much more than just a whim

Must work on myself, an example I'll be
Have patience, respect, truth and love, harmony

I can give him much more than money or wealth
A good, clean example will pass on good health

At some point I realized I might have to do some private counselling or therapy or whatever you want to call it to work on some issues that I needed to focus on. I met Clelia Costo who was giving a talk at the Serenity Shop in Vancouver and decided if I was going to work with anyone, it would be her. When I was ready I contacted her and we spent a few months doing weekly sessions. She helped me to clearly see what I needed to do. She helped me to solidify my healthy way of looking at myself and my life. Clelia was great but I think the key was I was ready to work on myself. I had peeled my "recovery onion" down to the point where I couldn't go back. I didn't want to go back. I had a real understanding of what had been going on in my life and I wasn't going to lie to myself anymore.

The thing that amazed me the most was the change that took place inside of me. You couldn't really see it on the outside except maybe by my different attitude. It was like I was a whole new person inside but the change came gradually over a long period of time.

Change is sometimes hard for people. Whatever is familiar is more comfortable even if that familiar is unhealthy. People are usually reluctant to change. They don't know how it will come out. They don't know what will happen. Fear of the unknown. But change is necessary for growth. Without it we stagnate.

Change

*Some people think the way they are is the way
    they'll always be,
But they don't realize there's a way that they
    can be set free*

*The answer doesn't come from taking all that
    you can get,
And you won't find the answer staring in your
    TV set*

*The answer isn't in a glass, a joint or in a pill,
The answer is already there, it's in your own
    free will*

*To look upon yourself as just a human, that
    is all
It doesn't matter if you're black or white, you're
    short or tall*

*We're all the same, we're human, then again,
    we're all unique,
There's lots of things that make us tick, there's
    many things we seek*

*We make mistakes, but just don't beat your head
    against the wall,
We learn from things that we do wrong, before
    we walk, we crawl*

*We take it one step at a time, we learn along
    the way,*
*We change the things we find don't work, we
    learn from every day*

*Yes, change can be a scary thing, but helps to
    let us grow,*
*It makes us better all the time, it puts us in
    the know*

*To change means life is always fresh, there's
    always something new,*
*I've changed some garbage in my life, I'm sure
    that you can too*

Spirituality

A Journey

Something I always had trouble with was the idea of God. I didn't know whether to believe or not. We weren't a church going family but what I did see of religion, I didn't like. In the news in Ireland, Catholics and Protestants were killing each other simply because of their religion. I read about Christian Missionaries and Crusaders who forced people to convert to their beliefs to be "saved". The more I learned about what different religious groups had done to each other through history, the more I disliked the idea of religion. The problem of course, was I was equating God with religion.

Before I go any further with the idea of God or rather spirituality, I am not in any way affiliated with any organized or unorganized religion. I don't go to church. I'm not going to tell you that you should believe this or believe that. You have the right to believe or not to believe anything you want. I would never tell you that you are wrong because of your beliefs. I am not a religious person. On the other hand, I consider myself a spiritual person.

For as long as I can remember, I've felt a deep connection with the Natural World. I believe that is where we came from. We are highly evolved animals from the Natural world. It seems to me, we don't like to look at ourselves as animals but that's what we are. God created us that way. Now you might say, "Hold on. You just contradicted yourself. You said we are highly evolved animals then you said God created us." Well, that's right. Why not? I believe in evolution and the God creation idea. I believe God created evolution.

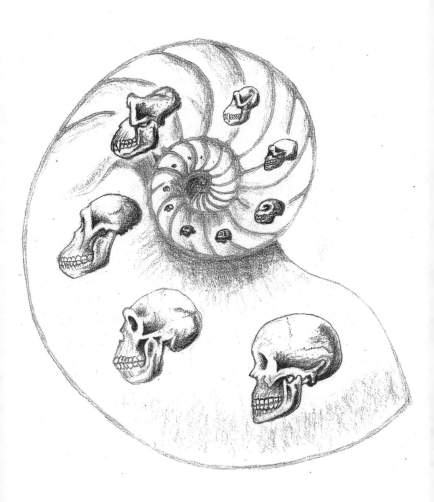

A Journey

Evolution is, in it's simplest form, the ability to adapt to change. Now, God created life on earth, why wouldn't He give his Creation the ability to adapt to change? In other words, to survive. It would have been a great waste of energy on God's part to create life on earth and then have it wiped out by some huge volcano or gigantic meteor. In my opinion, God created evolution and all life has been evolving ever since. Maybe that's why I've always felt comfortable in the Natural world. I believe that's where I came from. Walking through a forest is like a "religious" experience for me because I believe that's what my ancestors would have seen. I've always felt that I was related to every living thing. To me, it's like there is a universal energy that flows through all life. I used to say "I believe the energy that flows through a tree is the same energy that flows through me."

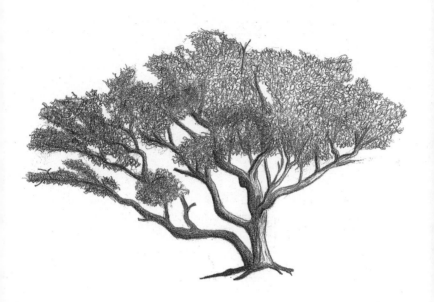

"In God We Trust"

"In God We Trust" boy, what a joke!
  At least it used to be.
For God and trust weren't in my life.
  It seemed that way to me.

How could there be a God, who leaves
  me feeling all this pain?
How could He be there when He lets
  abuse happen again?

How could there be a God when all
  those people have no food?
How could He be there and let all His
  people be so rude?

How could there be a God when people
  fight and kill and maim?
How could He be there when His people
  kill in His own name?

How could there be a God who lets
  the little babies die?
There's lots of thing I used to think,
  and then I'd heave a sigh.

"Hey! if you're real, come down and lift
  my bed or move my chair.
I don't trust that you're real at all,
  I don't believe you're there."

But that was then and this is now.
My thoughts are not the same.
I know that God is full of love.
It's Man who's filled with shame.

I trust now in the spirit that's alive
inside of me.
I know it's been there all the time,
it's just I didn't see.

Spirit

I don't have to go to church
To know I have a Higher Power
I don't have to be a sheep
To know I'll have my finest hour
I don't have to have someone
Tell me what my beliefs should be
I know that my beliefs are mine
What they are is up to me
And I believe there is a Spirit
That's alive in everything
It's in the plants and trees and worms
It's in the little birds that sing
It's in all forms of life
No matter if they're big or small
I feel the Spirit is in everyone
The Spirit is in us all

When I started to become involved in A.C.O.A., the subject of God was present. At first it bothered me but after a while, I realized I could interpret the word "God" any way I wanted to. I thought, "From now on, I'll just say that God is that universal energy. I can live with that."

People sometimes refer to God as their Higher Power. I started to accept the idea that there is something in the Universe higher up than we are.

After being in the recovery process for a while, I started to feel like I was being guided around. Like I was being taken to places I needed to be. It may sound funny but things just seemed to all fit together. It was like watching a three dimensional jigsaw puzzle put itself together right before my eyes. That's about the time I started writing poems. Sometimes they seemed to write themselves. It was almost like I wasn't really writing them, I was just writing them down.

Words

It's almost as if I hear words in my head
It's not like they're words that I've seen, heard or read
They seem to come from a place inside of me
They're wisdom, they're humour, they're sadness, they're free
I don't have to work, they just seem to be there
A continuous flowing of words I must bear
Sometimes I record them, like now, write them down
So I can re-live them, each verb, every noun
For when I preserve them for posterity
I realize a power is flowing through me
The spirit hath moved me, it's doing it now
I don't know just why and I'm not sure just how
But that doesn't matter, I'm glad that it's here
I'm humbled, and honoured and I have no fear
I trust that God will show me my destiny
I thank Him for what's been bestowed unto me

I couldn't explain what was really happening, but once I realized that "something" was happening, I would just be open to it and go with it. A classic example of that "something" happening is the poem "Change".

I was camping with my son in the Cariboo and I thought to myself when I get him to sleep, I'm going to write tonight. I was planning it. I even planned the subject. I was going to write about change. Actually, I wanted to write about it for my brother Lloyd. He was having some hard times in his life and I wanted to give him some inspiration. I wanted to help him see that change is possible, things don't have to be bad forever.

Anyway, I had a bit of trouble getting my son to go to sleep but, after he did, I sat down and tried to write. I tried really hard. I pushed and I wracked my brain but it just wasn't working. Finally, I got so frustrated that I said, "Forget it" and went to sleep.

About a week later, I was in the yard unloading planks off a flatdeck and I "heard" in my head "Some people think the way they are is the way they'll always be". I thought, "yeah, okay." Then I "heard": "But they don't realize there's a way that they can be set free". I thought, "Hey, I like that." Next, I "heard": "The answer doesn't come from taking all that you can get." And I actually said out loud, "Oh, no. It's starting..." I scrambled to find something to write it down on, while trying to remember what I was hearing. I found a dirty, crumpled up piece of paper and a dirty, old envelope. I frantically sharpened a big lumber pencil and within twenty minutes the poem "Change" poured out onto those two pieces of paper. I sat back exhilarated and said, "What the heck just happened?"

I still have those two dirty, crumpled up, scribbled on pieces of paper. I kept them because they're symbolic to me. To me, they represent being open and aware. Not being afraid to let things happen. Not being afraid to let go. If it feels right, run with it.

All I Can Do

All I can do is live for me,
I cannot live for you
I can't tell you what you should say,
or say what you should do
All I can do is do my best,
the best that I can be
To focus on the good in life,
and what is right for me

Whatever is right for me may not be right for you. I used to think, if it helps me then it will help you but I don't think that anymore. Everyone has their own path. What works for one person may not work for the next. Everyone is different. We all have our own ways of looking at things. We're all different yet we're all the same. I love the joke, "Remember, you are totally unique, just like everybody else."

This idea holds true for Spirituality. There are many ways of being spiritual and none of them, in my opinion, are wrong. If it brings you closer to your Higher Power, (however you want to interpret that), I think that's wonderful. I believe there is one God. There just happens to be a whole bunch of ways of getting in touch with Him or Her, if you prefer. I've heard people refer to God in the female sense. Why not? It's like the old saying "God is like a mountain. There are many paths that lead to the top."

That's the main problem I have with religions. Each one says "I'm right, you're wrong. And if you don't follow us you'll be spending Eternity in Hell." I hate it when people try to push their religion on you. Why can't all religions be right? Why would God set up a system where only a small select group of His children would be saved and everyone else would burn in Hell? Well, of course, He didn't. Man did. Man created religion. Man probably created the idea of Hell too, just to keep everybody in line.

It seems to me, the main motivation for many religions and churches has been the acquisition of power and money. Some religions actually dictate that you have to give up a certain percentage of your income to the church. I don't get the connection between spirituality and money. Money doesn't bring you closer to God. If anything, it probably takes you further away.

I don't care what religion you belong to or if you belong to one at all. It doesn't matter what your beliefs are. It doesn't matter to me what race you are, what colour you are, or what you look like. I just try to treat everybody the same. My philosophy is I try to treat people the way I would want them to treat me.

Do Unto Others

I try to live my daily life with one philosophy
To treat my fellow man the way I'd want them
to treat me
"Revenge is sweet" is not, to me, just what HE
had in mind
I don't think it's about revenge, it's about us
being kind
So every time I hear those words, they certainly
ring true
Do unto others as you would have them do unto you.

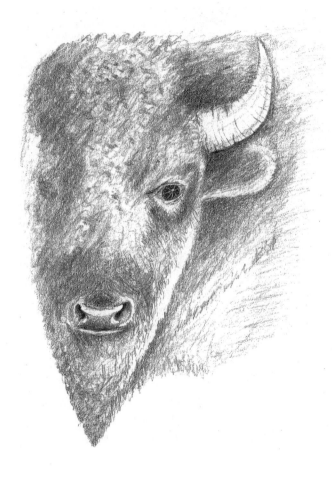

Native

A Journey

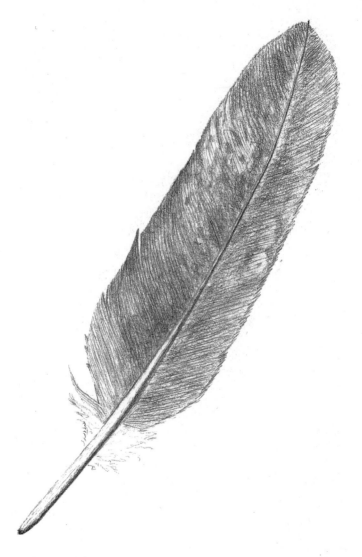

I mentioned before about my belief in a universal energy that flows through all living things. Because of that, I have always felt a connection to all peoples around the world. No matter what their race, that same energy is flowing through all of us. I have always been fascinated by indigenous peoples because they usually have their beliefs and culture deeply rooted in the natural world. They understand their place in nature because they are part of nature. They give respect to the rest of God's creation because their lives usually depend on it. They would take what they needed and leave the rest.

I feel especially connected to North American Natives. It seemed only natural when I met Phil L'Hirondelle in 1991. He ran a Native Indian bookstore called All My Relations on Granville Island in Vancouver. He also ran a Healing Circle once a week. A Healing Circle is a meeting facilitated by an Elder or Respected Person. There are some beginning ceremonies including the Smudge, a ritual smoke-cleansing, and then an eagle feather is passed around the Circle. Whoever is holding the feather becomes the Speaker and they can say anything they need to say. It's a safe, spiritual, non-judgmental environment. You can take your problems there and release them into the Circle. What amazed me about the Healing Circle was the similarities to an A.C.O.A. meeting. I realized Natives have been having support group meetings for a lot longer than we have.

The Circle

The fires burn
The wind will blow
The eagle flies
The rivers flow

The book of time
Turns one more page
Tobacco, sweet grass
Cedar, sage

The medicines of old
Are found
Within this circle
Turning round

The sacred flower
Of love can bloom
Within this safe
And chosen womb

The pain and hurt
Can be set free
Within this place
Of harmony

The love and joy
Is here to share
Within these walls
With those who care

The circle's here
For you and me
It will be for
Eternity

And if you're not
Sure where to start
Turn off your mind
Speak from your heart.

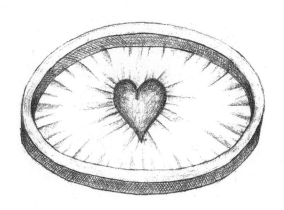

A Journey

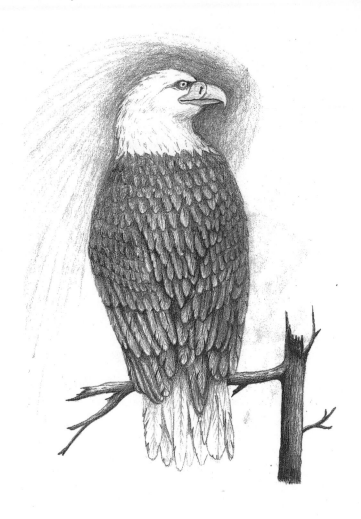

I began to learn more about Native Spirituality and developed a great respect for Native Culture. There is a strong belief in Native Culture that every living thing has a spirit, even non-living things. It seemed very similar to the way I have always viewed the natural world. There is, of course, God in Native Spirituality. There are many different words for God in different Native languages, but God is generally referred to as the Great Spirit.

After being involved in the Circle for a while I began to go to Sweat Lodges. A Sweat Lodge is also run by an Elder or Respected Person. It's essentially a dark steam sauna in which you pray. That may sound like a simple explanation but it is of course more involved than that. It is very spiritually enlightening. The general purpose of a Sweat is a physical, mental, emotional and spiritual cleansing.

Something else I was honoured to help out at was a Sun Dance. I didn't dance in the ceremony but I did bring up some supplies and help raise some tepees.

Through the Circle, the Sweat, the Sun Dance and my many conversations with Native people, I got to see the spiritual side of Native Culture. I got to see the healthy side. When I was growing up, all I ever heard about Indians was that they were drunks, bums, lazy and no good. Through my experiences, I got to see reality.

Cycles

All things come in cycles
Here on Mother Earth.
The cycles keep turning,
There's death and there's birth.
The time just keeps ticking
Creating a pace;
The world just keeps turning
Revolving in space.
It circles the sun
In exactly a year.
There's no myth or magic,
No reason for fear.
It's simply a cycle
Repeating again;
Don't know how it started,
We don't know just when.
The cycles keep turning
At all different speeds.
It depends on their size
Their shape and their needs.
The cycle of 24 hours
In a day.
Part of it's work
And part of it's play.
The cycle when people
Must bury their dead.
The cycle of losing
The hairs on your head.
The cycle of seeing a tree

Die and fall
And then see a tender
Young sapling grow tall.
The cycle that starts when a baby is born.
The cycle that ends
With the harvest of corn.
But then with that corn
A new cycle's begun –
It's picked and it's peeled
And it's dried in the sun.
It's cleaned and it's ground
And it's made into bread;
And yet a new cycle
When people are fed.
It seems that the cycles
Are all inter-wound.
They all seem connected,
They keep spinning round.
They keep this world moving,
They keep us alive.
They're what allows life
On this planet to thrive.
The death of a leaf
Means the birth of a worm.
We all need these cycles
On that I stand firm.
So take heart in knowing
That your life will end.
Remember, you're part
Of a cycle, my friend.

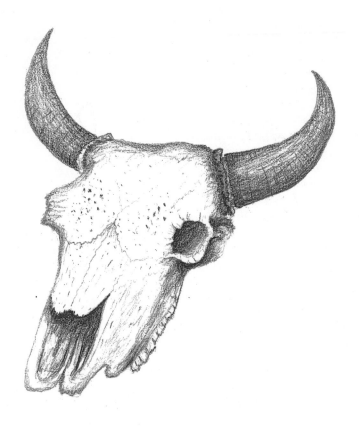

Death

As the old saying goes, "There are only two things you can be certain of in this world – death and taxes." Hopefully, we can get to the point somewhere in the future where we can eliminate taxes but we can never eliminate death. Not to say that mankind hasn't thought about it, written about it, or even dreamed about it. We would love to cheat death and achieve immortality. Even the idea of time travel is about death. If we could travel through time, we could cheat death. Essentially, time is death. If enough time passes by, eventually, we're all going to die.

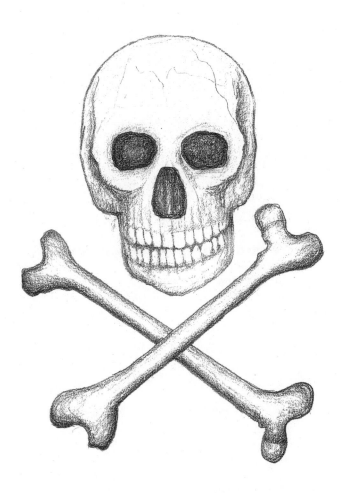

Life Is Short

*If there's one thing that I have learned, if there's one
thing I know*

*It's "Life Is Short" and there's no warning when it's
time to go.*

*You're here one minute, laughing, breathing, play-
ing, worry-free,*

*The next, you're gone. No second chance. That's it.
Eternity.*

*You could step off the curb one second faster than
you should*

*And get run down. You're D.O.A. Too bad. You're
gone for good.*

*It could be cancer, lightning, earthquake, flood or
even fire.*

*The thought of taking my last breath's not some
thing I desire.*

*It doesn't matter how you go, the end result's the
same.*

*It's not a minor penalty. You're thrown out of the
game.*

*Now please don't think I'm morbid, coming up with
ways to die –*

*The point is I don't want to go. Don't want to say
good-bye.*

*I've got too much I haven't done, too much I want to
do,*

*Please God don't take me yet because we know that
I'm not through.*

*I haven't ended War. I haven't cured the common
cold.*

I haven't found a way to turn grass clippings into gold.
I haven't rid the world of hatred, waste and crime and greed.
I haven't solved the hunger problem or the housing need.
I haven't stopped pollution and I haven't saved the whale
Or harnessed fusion energy or found the Holy Grail.
I'm not done yet. There's lots more work that's left that must be done.
I'll do my best to save the world and then I'll have some fun.

A Journey

Obviously a bit of tongue in cheek there, but the idea is "Don't waste your time". There's so much to do and so little time. One of the things I've thought about and don't want to see happen is to be laying on my death bed, about to pass away, and say "Damn, I didn't finish this and I never got to that and I'm not going to have a chance to do that other thing". I don't want to have any big regrets when I pass on to the next level.

But people do pass on to the next level. They do die. Actually, we don't seem to like the words "die" and "dead". We say it in all sorts of poetic, flowery ways that sound more colourful and less permanent. Passed away. Passed on. Gone to meet his maker. Pushing up daisies. Bit the big one. He's not with us anymore. Eternal sleep. Safe in the arms of God. Deceased. Went to the great beyond. Sold the farm. Playing cards with St. Peter. Gone to the big _____ in the sky. (That's one you can personalize, If the person was a baker, you could say "Gone to the big bakery in the sky.") Up in heaven. Walking through the Pearly Gates. Taking harp lessons. Looking down on us. Watching over us. With the angels now. God needed an angel. Has gone towards the light. The list could go on and on.

We have trouble accepting death for what it is. It's death. For whatever reason, the end of life. Some deaths are what we would call "normal". My maternal grandmother lived to be 80 years old. Her mind was still very active but her body just couldn't take it anymore. While she was hospitalized, she had a series of complications and passed away. Or should I say she died. Essentially due to old age. That's what we would call a "normal" death. People get old, they die. "Normal".

My paternal grandmother never got to become old. Through no fault of her own, she couldn't handle the pain, stress and abuse in her life. She committed suicide by drinking a bottle of Lysol. "Not normal". I never got to meet her. She died before I was even born.

My father died of a heart attack at the age of 50. Even though he wasn't old, as in elderly, he was at a high risk of having a heart attack. He was overweight, he drank, took up smoking after quitting for 10 years, and was under a huge amount of stress. Even though 50 isn't old, his death is somewhat "normal" considering the conditions in his life. People can be killed in any number of ways and at any age. Those deaths are considered unnatural – "not normal". A death becomes glaringly "not normal" when a child dies. Especially when it's your own child. If you're a parent, you've probably thought about it, and then quickly erased it from your mind. It couldn't happen to you, right? It's always the "other" guy who suffers the tragedy. That's what I thought until my two young sons drowned in a pool. Luckily, they were able to revive and save my oldest son but my youngest wasn't so lucky. It's every parents' worst nightmare. It's the hardest thing I've ever had to face. I pray I'll never have to face it again. It's the ultimate pain.

The Ultimate Pain

I feel so many different pains
They're all deep down inside
But one pain's greater than them all
The one since Thomas died

You really can't imagine
The things that you go through
When instantly your little love
Is snatched away from you

You can't say "STOP! Just go away
This isn't happening"
When all the words the doctors say
So loudly do they ring

"I think the four year old will make it
I think we got him quick
But, oh, that little two year old
He's really very sick"

"His heart, it stopped, for half an hour
We finally got it going
But I'm afraid the pressure in his head
Is quickly growing"

"His brain is swelling
From the lack of oxygen, you see
And there's about a zero chance
That he'll ever be three"

I wish I could just pick him up
And give him a big hug
I never thought on my own child
I'd have to pull the plug

I know it's best, his brain is flat
There's no activity
His soul's in heaven, there's only
His body here with me

The pain, the pain, it chews me up
And spits me out again
But now I know by feeling it
The healing can begin

There's other pain I feel besides
The pain of losing Thomas
Abuse, neglect, abandonment
But now I know there's promise

There's hope that just by being real
And feeling what is here
I find that pain is natural
Not something I should fear

It helps me cope, to understand
That it's OK to mourn
For pain is just a part of life
It starts the day we're born

❦

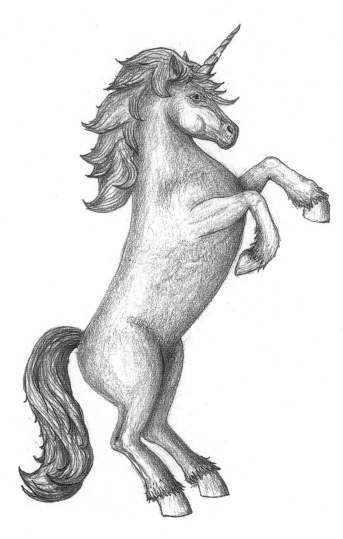

Death, sometimes, can be cruel. It can be mean. It can be ugly. It can seem very unfair but we need death. Without death, there is no life. We have to accept that death is "normal" because life is fragile. We have to take care of ourselves. You never know when you're gonna go.

Actually, I plan on dying on my 85th birthday. I do things rather slowly and I figure I should be able to get most of my work done by then.

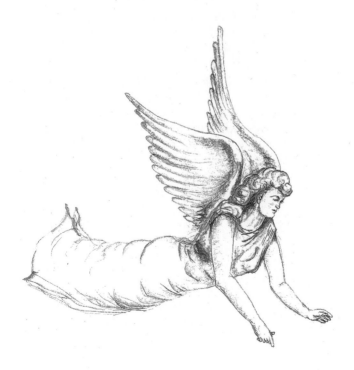

Death

I used to feel uncomfortable
When thinking about death
For when you're dead, your life is done
It ends with your last breath
But now I see that death
Is not as final as I thought
Your body dies, yes, that is true
But that's not all you've got
You have a soul, and that lives on
For all eternity
Now I am not afraid of death
It doesn't bother me
For when my time has come to die
And when my life is done
I'll get to go to heaven
And I'll get to see my son

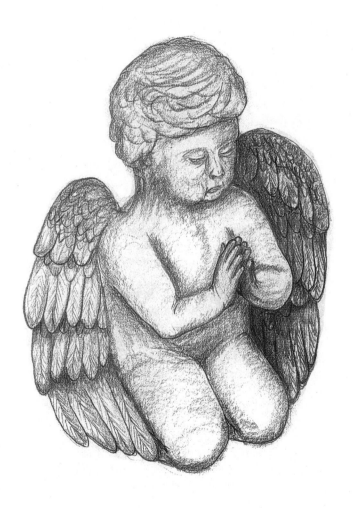

Another person in my life who has died a "not normal" death, is my brother Lloyd. His death was very "not normal". He didn't die accidentally or get really sick. He was murdered. A man who was staying at Lloyd's house shot him in the heart. He then proceeded to roll his body in a carpet, tie it up with rope, drive him up a mountain road outside of Squamish, B.C., then dispose of Lloyd's body by throwing it over a 600 foot cliff. Definitely very "not normal".

One of the interesting aspects of Lloyd's case was, we didn't know what happened to him. He became a missing person.

When someone dies, let's say in a car accident, you know what happened. They're dead. Unless it's an unusual car accident, you can probably figure out who's fault it was, if anyone's. Then deal with the circumstances and get on with the grieving process. That's a very important part of the cycle of life and death. Being able to grieve the loss of a loved one. But when someone goes missing, you don't know if you should grieve or not. Are they dead? Did they run away? Do they have amnesia and have just wandered off? Are they in South America or is their body in a ditch somewhere? You just don't know.

At this point, I'd like to say my heart goes out to all the people and families who have missing loved ones out there. I do have "some" idea what it's like.

Lloyd was my brother but, for my Mom, Lloyd was her child, her son, her baby. When someone is missing, you're in limbo. You're just hanging there.

You're just waiting, wondering; and wait we did.
Lloyd was missing for two years when his skeletal
remains were found by a hiker. Then of course
WHAM!! You're no longer in limbo. You don't have
to wonder if he's dead or alive. Now you know.

But then a whole new set of questions comes up.
What happened? How the hell did his body get
halfway up a mountain rolled in a carpet? Who did
this? Why did they do this? Are we ever going to find
out who did it?

The missing person investigation moved to a
murder investigation. A year later a man was
charged with Second Degree Murder for Lloyd's
death. He eventually pleaded guilty to Manslaughter
and got four years in jail. To us, it doesn't seem like
enough but what can you do?

Now, I'm not going to go into all the details here
about Lloyd's murder although it's a very interesting
case. It's a whole book in itself. The prosecutor told
me it's just about the strangest case she's ever dealt
with.

Why?

There never seems to be an answer to the question: Why?
It never seems to make much sense when loved ones up
and die.
Why'd he have to die? God should have taken me
instead.
He was so young. I've lived my life. It should be me that's
dead.
Why'd he have to work so hard and strain his weakened
heart?
Why do I feel guilty when I know I did my part?
Why'd she have to go so fast? I didn't say goodbye.
Why's she gone? It's just not fair! She wouldn't hurt a
fly.
Why'd he go and get that drunk and think that he could
drive?
Why'd we fight so bad the last time I saw him alive?
Why'd he kill him? Why'd they fight? Why is my brother
dead?
Why? Oh why? All the unanswered whys still fill my head.
But then I guess there's some things we're not supposed
to know.
Why was I born? Why am I here? Why will I have to go?
We're not in charge. We can't control the Who, What,
When and Why.
I guess when someone goes that it was just their time to
die.

ॐ

Lloyd

A Journey

Something interesting happened when I started writing about my brother, Lloyd. I realized I was still angry with him. Lloyd and I were very different. Although we looked very similar, we were like night and day. He was the loud, aggressive, hyper one. I was the quiet, passive, relaxed one. Throughout most of our lives, we were like opposing forces. Sibling rivalry for sure. But there were a few things that we shared. I know we both loved each other. We frustrated and exasperated each other but underneath that I know we cared a lot for one another. It was just hard to bring that to the surface. You know, that "man stuff". Keep your feelings pushed down.

We also shared an interest in alcohol and drugs, I preferred marijuana. He preferred cocaine. Our choice in drugs matched our personality types. Pot slows you down, cocaine speeds you up.

I truly believe that something else we shared was a low self-esteem. Two people can have exactly the same problem but manifest it in totally different ways. When someone feels helpless and out of control, they may take on the "victim" role. They may feel that they have no power and everyone is pulling their strings. They feel useless. Someone else who also feels helpless and out of control may take on the "aggressor" role. They may feel that their life is out of control so, to correct that, they have to control everything and everyone else. That way, they gain back the stability they need by feeling like they are "in charge". Same problem, just different ways of dealing with it. Both of them unhealthy.

Now, I'm not going to sit here and trash my brother and his memory. I'm not going to rattle off a list of things I think he did wrong but, I' m also not going to sugar-coat the whole thing and say we had a wonderful, warm relationship. We used to fight, physically and verbally. I used to get very angry with him. I did things that I regret. I'm sure there are some things he regretted but we all have problems. We all make mistakes. We all have things that we could have done differently. I think that's why I was most angry at Lloyd. He didn't deal with some small problems. He let them turn into big ones which ultimately contributed to his demise. Not to say that the person who murdered Lloyd isn't responsible for his death. Of course, he is. But if Lloyd would have changed the path that he was on, I believe, that he would still be alive today.

It's easy to deny you have a problem. The hard part is admitting you have one and doing something about it. None of us like to admit we have faults but if we ignore them long enough, they can turn into really BIG problems.

It's possible Lloyd's decision making processes were affected by head injuries he may have received in two separate motor vehicle accidents in his life. A psychiatrist also diagnosed him as having Attention Deficit Disorder.

Lloyd really needed help and I tried to offer him my support. I told him about what had been helping me and offered to take him to a support group meeting. He was very receptive and seemed enthusiastic at first but, as the weeks went by, he kept coming up with excuses of why he couldn't go. Then, finally, he rejected the whole idea. We had a fight one night and he said "That's YOU and YOUR stuff. It has nothing to do with me." Another time he also said "I don't have a problem with my drinking, YOU have a problem with my drinking." I really wanted to help Lloyd but it got to the point where I couldn't help him if he didn't want to help himself. I had to kind of step away and take care of myself.

It's hard for me to write about Lloyd. My mind goes in six different directions at the same time. We had great times together. We had really bad times together. We always loved each other but sometimes, we hated each other. Sometimes he was my best friend; other times, my worst enemy. Sometimes he was his OWN worst enemy. I'm trying to be respectful. Lloyd's not here to defend himself. I really wish he was here. I miss him. He was my brother. But, I'm also trying to be honest. I'm not going to lie to myself about the past. Sometimes it wasn't very pretty. I'm just trying to be truthful.

The Truth

If asked to state my highest moral value,
then I'd say

I tell the truth in everything,
I live it every day

I used to lie to hide my shame and
cover up my act

But then it became very hard to tell
the fib from fact

One lie leads to another and before
you know...you're caught

A lie exposed became the source of
many battles fought

But I have learned dishonesty will
only bring you down

No longer will I play the fool or
have to be the clown

I cannot and I will not lie
I hate dishonesty

The truth be known...the truth's the
most important thing to me

Dear Lloyd,

You always had something to do.
I didn't spend much time with you.

You always had somewhere to go.
You often said, "Hey, later Bro."

And you went your way; I went mine.
"I'll see you later", that was fine.

But now it's later – you're not here.
You won't be back; that's crystal clear.

I'll never hear that laugh again.
I'll have to just remember when

We went to Reno, Vegas too,
And all the crazy things we'd do.

The way that we both bugged each other.
The way that we both loved our mother.

No matter if we lost or won,
We were just out to have some fun.

The joy and pain all through the years,
The laughter, smiles and all the tears.

Now, all I have are memories.
God take this message, would you please?

Please take this message, way up high;
I never got to say good-by.

Good-by Lloyd. I love you.
>   *Your "Bigger Little" Brother*
>   *Randy*

Be Kind

Something that often seems to be hard for us, is to be kind to ourselves. It's always easier to help some needy person, volunteer for some cause, work overtime, help someone move, take a sick friend flowers or just be there for someone else. What about being there for ourselves.

For most of my life, it felt strange and uncomfortable doing positive, healthy things for myself. Usually, I didn't do them. It felt more natural doing unhealthy things because it matched how I felt about myself. I didn't feel worthy of being happy and healthy. I didn't think I deserved a good life so I made bad choices for myself.

I believe the most powerful low self-esteem reinforcer is how we talk to ourselves inside our own heads. Negative mind talk. It used to seem like my mind would never "shut up". Always telling me what a jerk I was, what a failure I was, what an idiot I was. Reminding me I didn't deserve "this" and I didn't deserve "that". If I encountered a healthy, self-assured, confident person my mind would make sure I got as far away from that person as possible. Healthiness intimidated me. I was uncomfortable with people thanking me or complimenting me. I would minimize it or make some excuse about how it wasn't as good as they thought. Compliments are good. Good is healthy. Healthy is uncomfortable. So, push it away.

Once I realized how damaging negative mind talk could be to your self-esteem, I began to recognize it and face it when it came up. I would short circuit the negative mind talk by telling myself the opposite. It was very strange for a while because there was a constant battle going on inside my head. The negative mind talk was so well-rooted and flowed so easily, that it took quite some time to really get a handle on it. But soon, I was able to instantly recognize the negative and immediately counter-act it. Eventually the negative mind talk was replaced by positive thoughts and feelings. I now know that I am a worthy, honest, humble, positive, likable, intelligent, talented human being. I am very thankful for all the experiences in my life, good and bad. All those experiences are gifts that have been given to me to help me grow as a person.

I used to compare my life to other people's lives and wish I had the things that they did. Their lives always looked better than mine. But comparing yourself to others can be a dangerous thing. We are all different. We are all unique in our own ways. I'm just thankful for being here.

Thankful

I'm glad that I am thankful
When I look at what I've got
I used to see what others had
And then what I had not
I've changed the way I see the world
And everything within
No longer do I look at life
As something that you win
There always will be someone
That will have more things than you
But dwelling on what others have
Is not the thing to do
For envy gets you nowhere
And it's not the thing for me
I'm glad that I am thankful
And that's how I want to be

I've had a lot of painful things happen in my life. I wouldn't want to have to go through them again, but if I could wave a magic wand and change those experiences, I wouldn't change anything. All those events in my life have contributed to the person I am today. I like myself now. I'm proud of myself. I wouldn't want to change that.

I am a worthy human being and so are YOU.

So, tell yourself positive things. Be good to yourself. Treat yourself fairly. Don't beat yourself up especially over mistakes. Mistakes are good. Mistakes are how we learn. Mistakes make us better people by telling us what not to do. Tell yourself nice things like:

My opinion does count.
I have good ideas.
It's okay to change my mind.
I have a right to my opinion.
I have a right to be here.
I have the ability to change.
I want to improve the things I don't like about
    myself.
I want to be healthy.
I choose to do the right thing.
I have the right to make healthy choices for myself.
It's okay to distance myself from people who are
    abusive towards me.
You can't make me do something I don't want to do.

It makes me feel good to help people but I won't help
someone at my own expense.

I will not be afraid to say how I feel.

I won't be afraid to be who I am: Me.

I will not lie to myself.

I enjoy taking myself to healthy places.

I won't beat myself up for mistakes I've made in the
past.

I love and accept myself.

I will not allow people to push my buttons.

I am thankful for what I have.

I will take care of myself because I'm worth it.

I deserve to be treated with respect.

No one has the right to abuse me.

I will not let anyone squash my dreams.

I will live my life the way I want.

I deserve the good things in life.

I understand and accept my past.

I accept I cannot change the past.

I willingly take on the responsibility of making my
future a healthier place to live.

I will allow myself to have fun.

I accept and embrace the childlike qualities within
me.

I am trustworthy.

I am honest.

I am a good person.

I will not blame myself for other people's mistakes.
I will not take on someone else's responsibilities.
I will take responsibility for my own actions.
I want what is best for me.
I will not belittle another human being.
I will not let someone else belittle me.
I will do something nice for myself today.
I will do something nice for someone else today.
I deserve to be happy.
I like who I am.
I am thankful for all the lessons that have been
        given to me.
I believe in myself.

In the beginning it might seem strange to be saying positive things to yourself. If you're like me and have many years of negative mind talk, it may take a while before you become comfortable with positive mind talk. It doesn't even matter if you believe it or not at first. The important thing is to recognize how damaging the negative talk is and replace it with the positive. Whatever negative thoughts come up, say to yourself something like "No, I'm not going to do that to myself anymore. I won't listen to it. I deserve better than that." Just keep saying healthy things to yourself and after a while, you WILL believe them because they are true. You ARE a worthy human being. No one has the right to treat you badly. Not even YOU. Okay, you do have that right but it's not a healthy choice.

I Release Myself

It seems that I've been carrying
A load that isn't mine
A crime's committed by someone
But then I pay their fine
Can't take responsibility
For their own acts of shame
'Someone' must be responsible
So then 'I' took the blame
But that is it, the time has come
I know I've had enough
They'll have to stand up for themselves
They'll have to face their stuff
"I hereby do release myself"
"From all their shame and guilt"
I won't let someone else's crap
Destroy what I have built

Dear You,

Be nice to yourself. Be kind to yourself. Don't strive for perfection. Perfection is boring. Be real. Be who you are. You are enough just the way you are. You don't have to be something you're not. Allow yourself to take risks. Through risks come rewards. Be honest with yourself. Be responsible for your own actions. Allow others to be responsible for their actions. Don't feel that you have to 'rescue' everyone. Don't allow other people to pull you down. Stand up and be proud of who you are.

Sincerely,
Me

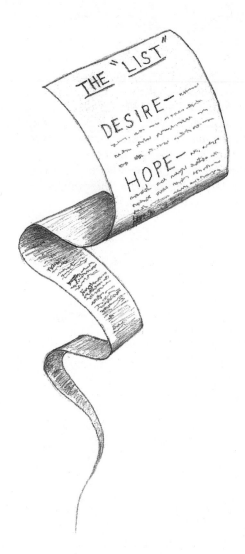

The "List"

I've had people say things to me like "It sounds like you've struggled with the same things I'm struggling with. Low self-esteem, abuse, addiction. What did you do? What can I do?"

Unfortunately we live in a fast paced society. Everything whizzes here and zooms there. We want everything to happen RIGHT NOW. We get upset when we have to wait 30 seconds at a traffic light. As a society, we are not very patient. We don't like to wait. We want the answer NOW. We want the "quick fix".

I believe, when it comes to the concept of recovery, there is no "quick fix". Things take time. It took a long time to get all screwed up. It will take a while to get "un"-screwed up.

When I sat down and really thought about what I had done, I realized that, over a period of time, I had developed a list of sorts. A list of ways of thinking. States of mind. Ways of looking at things and events that were different than the way I used to perceive them.

I'll try to run through the list with a brief explanation of what each one means to me. First of all, and I believe most important is:

Desire or wanting: A desire to be healthy. A desire for change. Wanting to have a better life.

Willingness: To be willing to change for the better. To be willing to make sacrifices and go through uncomfortable times. To be willing to be vulnerable. Willing to take risks.

Patience: To know that it takes time. To know that things aren't going to change overnight. To not give up just because it isn't easy.

Faith: To have faith that things will get better. Faith in a power greater than ourselves.

Trust: Trust in yourself. Trust that you're a good person. Trust that you can make good, healthy choices.

Honesty: Being honest with yourself. Facing the truth and not backing down from it. Admitting to yourself that you have problems that need to be worked on.

Forgiveness: Forgiving yourself for the mistakes and bad choices you've made in the past. Forgiving the people who have hurt you, if not verbally, at least in your own mind and realizing that they have had their own problems too.

Perseverance: Sticking with it no matter how uncomfortable it gets. Don't give up – keep trying.

Humility: Being humble enough to keep your ego from stopping your progress. Being modest.

Humanity: Realizing you are part of the human race. Feeling a sense of belonging in being human. Being humane to yourself, people around you, and all living things.

Realism: Being realistic in your expectations of yourself and the world around you. Don't set goals for yourself that are difficult or impossible to achieve. Don't set yourself up to fail.

Hope: Holding on to a sense that everything can and will improve.

Strength: Being aware of your inner strength and drawing on it when necessary.

Openness: Being open to new ideas and thoughts. Openness is the key to learning. A closed mind can't let in any new ideas.

Objectivity: To remain optimistic about your chances for improvement and success. Being optimistic that you can have a healthy future.

Compassion: Compassion for yourself and those around you. Admitting that what you have gone through has been very hard.

Assertiveness: Assert your right to be treated with respect. Defend yourself. Don't allow others to walk all over you. Positively state and maintain your position.

Non-judgmental: Being accepting of other people realizing that they have as much a right to be here as you do. What right do I have to judge anyone?

Empathy: Truly try to see something from another person's perspective. Put yourself in someone else's shoes and then re-think the situation.

Acceptance: Accepting yourself as a worthy human being. Accepting that you can't change the past. Accepting other people for who they are.

Love: Loving yourself and people around you.

Realizing that you are worthy of being loved by others.

Awareness: Being aware of the world around you. Being aware of your feelings and actions. Just being aware.

Responsibility: Being responsible for your own actions. Not trying to pass the buck or blame someone else for something you're responsible for.

Now I'm not going to say that I live this list every minute, every day. Or that I have the whole list down pat. I struggle with these items too. I'm a human being just like you. Sometimes it's hard to assert myself or forgive someone or be patient or be objective or trust or be open, but I try. I'm aware. I do my best. I realize that these are good qualities to have and I embrace them. I enjoy them.

My life used to be the opposite of everything on that list. I'm truly thankful that I stuck with it and didn't fall back into denial. It wasn't easy. It took a long time. There wasn't any "quick fix". No magic pill. Just be honest with yourself and have faith in yourself. There's help out there. You'll find it if you look for it.

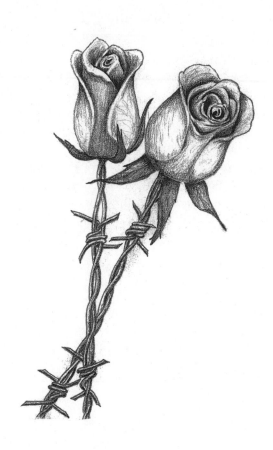

Memories

A Journey

Memories are funny things. A good memory can make you feel warm all over and put a smile on your face. A bad memory can put you in a deep depression. What are memories anyway? In a very clinical sense, memories are simply the brain's ability to record and store events in your life. It's like we all have our own super-computers between our ears. It can store your entire lifetime of events and experiences in its memory banks. The human brain is an amazing thing. Even though we know more about it now than we ever did before, we still don't know everything about how the brain works. The brain stores memories but it also records emotions and feelings. Different stimuli like sights, sounds and even smells can trigger hidden memories. The brain can sometimes throw us a curve ball by bringing up memories, thoughts and feelings at seemingly strange times. Memories can be triggered by any number of things.

I personally have had trouble with my memory. Actually my memory is great, it's just that my recall factor isn't so good. Sometimes I need a trigger to be able to recall a certain memory. There are, however, a lot of things I can't remember. There are periods in my childhood that are blank.

When events and experiences are painful, the brain sometimes blocks out certain memories and time periods as a sort of defense mechanism. By blocking out those memories, the brain is trying to protect you from having to go through those experiences all over again. I understand the process but I don't know if that's always such a good idea. Although events and times in my life have been painful and uncomfortable, I've learned from them and they've helped contribute to who I am today.I don't want to constantly relive them but I accept all the bad times in my life because they've helped me to appreciate the good times. If I didn't see the ugliness, it would be more difficult to truly appreciate the beauty. I'm thankful for all the pain in my life because it has helped me to be able to really feel the joy. It may sound paradoxical and I guess it is but it's really all about balance. You have to be able to see both sides so you know where the middle is. Even though some of my memories aren't all that pleasant, that's okay. They're my memories. I can't change them. They are things that have happened to me. They're a part of my life. I can't change the past. I have to accept it. Memories are my past. When it comes right down to it, memories are all we really have. We can acquire nice material things and try to be comfortable in this life but the only thing we truly have are our memories. Everything else can be taken away. So hold on to your memories. They're precious.

Precious

Sometimes the things that mean so much
Are things that we can't see or touch.

Sometimes they're worth much more than gold
And you can keep them 'til you're old.

Although they're priceless, you will see
They can't be bought, for they are free.

They're special moments, special ways
That life unfolds throughout your days.

They're good times and they're bad times too.
They're all the things that you've been through.

They're who you are and why you're here.
They're every smile. They're every tear.

Don't lose them. They can't be replaced.
To wipe them out would be a waste.

So don't forget them. Keep them. Please.
They're precious: They're your memories.

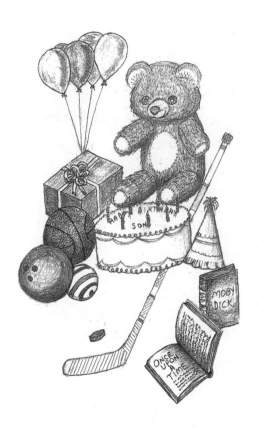

A Journey

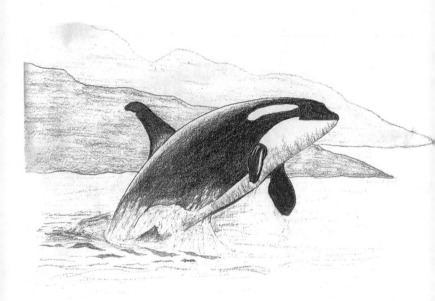

The World

Once I had a handle on myself, I started looking around. I saw the world in a whole new light. I could appreciate things a lot more. I realized it's all in how you look at it. It's all in your perception. Beauty is in the eye of the beholder.

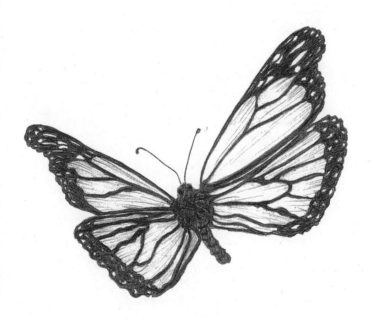

The World's Full Of Beauty

The world's full of beauty
The world's filled with pain
The world's warmed by sunshine
And soaked down by rain

If you look for beauty
You'll find it no doubt
The world's full of beauty
It's what life's about

But seek out what's painful
You will find that too
Just sit there and worry
And fret, steam and stew

Yes, everyone's problems
Will climb on your back
And if you allow it
You'll always get flack

They'll dump on you here
And they'll dump on you there
It doesn't seem right
And that's true, it's not fair

You'll find what you seek
Whether beauty or pain
The world's full of beauty
I've said it again

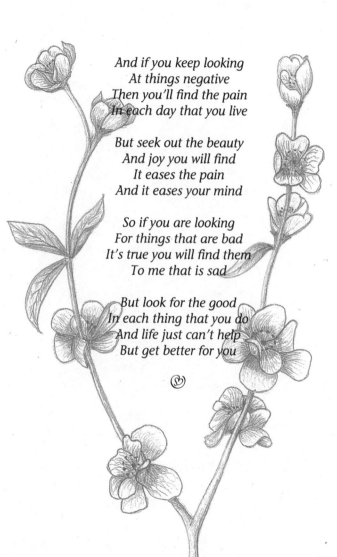

And if you keep looking
At things negative
Then you'll find the pain
In each day that you live

But seek out the beauty
And joy you will find
It eases the pain
And it eases your mind

So if you are looking
For things that are bad
It's true you will find them
To me that is sad

But look for the good
In each thing that you do
And life just can't help
But get better for you

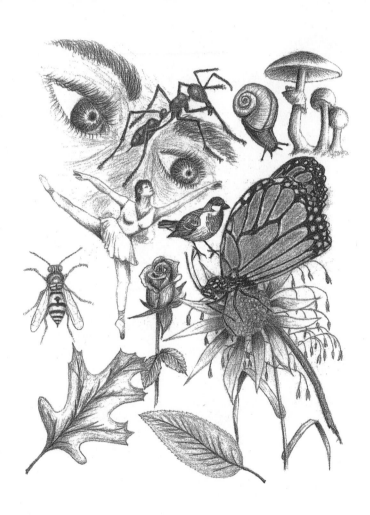

I See The Beauty

If you keep up a hectic pace
You'll miss the beauty of this place.
For in the past I didn't see
The beauty that surrounded me.
I used to run through every day,
I didn't "live" along the way.
I just did not appreciate
That good things come to those who wait.
Now I see beauty everywhere
It's in the clouds, it's in the air.
There's beauty in a blade of grass;
There's beauty in a dancing class.
I see beauty in trees and plants –
I see it in the wasps and ants.
There's beauty in the creeks and streams;
There's beauty in your thoughts and dreams.
I see the beauty in your face –
I see it in the Human Race.
I see beauty in death and birth.
I see it in our Mother Earth.
So take your time. You'll see. It's there –
Just look. There's beauty EVERYWHERE.

A Journey

When you're absorbed in your routine, whether it's rushing to the office, going to the bar, taking care of the kids, going to school or whatever, we tend to see the big things and miss the little things. There's so much going on around us that we sometimes put on blinders and only focus on one thing. We get to the point where nothing else seems to matter. There's a lot going on out there.

I remember there was a lady I used to know who often talked about her dog. She had a German Shepherd and would relate stories of how the dog would keep her company and was always there for her. She really loved that dog. She always reminded me of the beauty and comfort that is to be found by keeping in touch with the animal world.

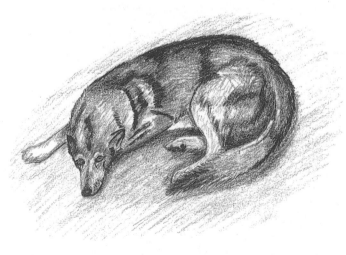

It's A Dog's Life

It's almost sad, they grow so fast
You wish the puppy stage could last
They're cute and bouncy, soft and fun
Endless energy, jump and run
They'll lick your face and nip your nose
Chew your socks and bite your toes
They love to play, to scrap and bark
They've always got that zest, that spark
And even when that pup gets old
It's heart stays young, won't treat you cold
But most of all, they're loyal and true
Won't cause you pain like people do
They're always glad to see your face
They're not constantly on your case
They let you live the way you want
Won't torture, tease, cause hurt and taunt
Just give them food, a place to sleep
A joyous bond you both shall reap
They do play games, but you will find
It's with a stick, and not your mind

Chance Meeting

I'm watching her
She's watching me
She turns away so gracefully
She's beautiful in every way
I wish that she would only stay
I'd love to spend more time with her
She's really set my heart astir
But I know that we're worlds apart
Even though she has touched my heart
I'm all alone, she's walked away
But of that moment I must say
I'm glad we were together here
But I'm a man, and she's a deer

Once, when I was up at my aunt and uncle's cattle ranch in Sorrento, it was calving time and there were some newborn calves settling in with their mothers. It was time for another calf to be born but it was a breech birth. The mother was having a lot of trouble. My uncle tried for hours to help her along but by the time the calf was born, it had died. I was standing there looking at this tiny, lifeless little calf. Then I thought of the other little calves who were with their mothers and I realized that death is a part of life. You can't have just one side. Everything has to balance out.

The World Is In Balance

In death there is life
The circle comes round
The World is in balance
In silence there's sound

There's opposite sides
To each thing on this Earth
For when there is death
There most surely is birth

You can't have just one part
You must accept both
For if you're one sided
You'll surely stunt growth

Each thing has its place
God made it that way
There's winter and summer
There's night and there's day

There's evil and angels
There's good and there's bad
Sometimes you are happy
And sometimes you're sad

You may not agree with
All things that I say
But the World is in balance
God made it that way

This world we live in is a wondrous place. It's full of miracles and amazing things but this world is also a very fragile place. Mankind has an awesome and daunting responsibility. We have the ability to destroy this planet. Wait a minute. Let me correct that. A native elder once told me that man is arrogant to think he can destroy this planet. He can't but he can kill all the life on it. We have to take care of this place. As far as we know this is the only planet in the universe where life exists. Personally, I'm sure there is other life forms out there somewhere but we don't know that for sure. It would be a real shame to destroy our only home.

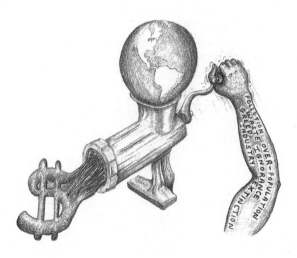

Help

I send a plea to Outer Space
To come and help the Human Race
We're having trouble on our own
We're headed for destruction zone

We're taking way more than our share
Most people just don't seem to care
We treat each other like we're dirt
It seems mankind is full of hurt

We've raped our home, destroyed our land
We've turned our topsoil into sand
Pollute our waters, kill our trees
Men seem to do just what they please

Without a thought of what they leave
This madness is hard to believe
How could Man be so ignorant
We're not Earth's only occupant

There's birds and insects, animals too
But Man locks them up in a zoo
There's trees and plants, whales and fish
To sum it up...I have one wish

If Man can't change his evil way
Then down upon my knees I pray
That we get help from up above
To help us change our hate to love

To show respect to living things
To see the balance that life brings
But help won't come from Outer Space
We'll find that in God's loving face

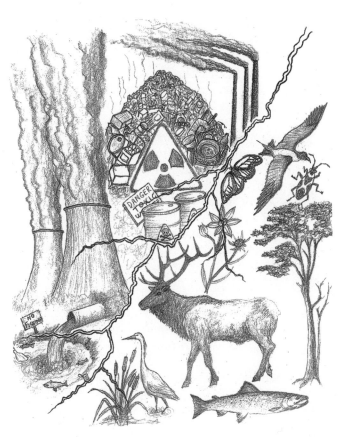

I hate waste! There's not too many things in this world that I can honestly say I hate but waste is one of them. Modern society is extremely wasteful. We don't even really have to work at it. We just seem to waste things naturally. Paper, food, water, energy, time, resources – you name it, we'll find a way to waste it. In North America, I think we are especially wasteful because we seem to take everything for granted. We don't really appreciate how well off we are. Scores of people from other countries would line up just to get into our garbage dumps. Most of us blindly run through our lives without really thinking about the consequences of our actions. Whatever we don't need at that moment, we trash it. It's so easy to just throw it away, toss it out or flush it without thinking about what happens to it after that. We've developed a system that keeps chewing things up and spitting them out. We truly are a "Throw Away Society". It's embarrassing really, the amount of garbage we produce every year.

I'm glad to see the increase in recycling lately but a lot more is needed. More emphasis needs to be put on recycling efficiently as in what we recycle something back into. For example, if we recycle clean white paper and turn it back into white paper again, there's not loss there. But if we take clean white paper and recycle it into egg cartons or fast food drink trays, then we downgrade to a less desirable end product.

Something I was shocked to see a few years ago was what happens to recycled glass. Not to say that this happens all the time but I saw truck loads of crushed glass, green, brown and clear being used as backfill around the foundation of a new high rise building. I had always thought that glass was recycled back into glass again. Now, granted, all that glass didn't end up in a landfill site but it just ended up being buried somewhere else. This opened my eyes to the fact that not everything gets recycled efficiently. I guess not every city has all the industry required to properly recycle all its materials. So, what can we do? Either build better recycling facilities or become less wasteful. How about both?

There are thousands of ways we can become more efficient and less wasteful. Manufacturers are starting to respond to the demand for less packaging. The sheer waste in packaging is horrendous. How many times have you brought something home from the store, opened the box, and then had to fight through layers of cardboard, paper, plastic and styrofoam? Then you've got a big pile of stuff you have to throw away. What about cereal boxes? What do we need a box for? There's already a bag inside. Why don't we just print all the information on the bag? I could rattle off a whole list of ways that manufacturers could be less wasteful and I'm sure you could too. I for one, would be more willing to buy something if it had less packaging.

Years ago, I had an idea for a non-profit organization called P.O.W.E.R. It stood for People Outraged at Wasting Earth's Resources. It would be a Waste Watchdog. Members would always be on the look out for any kind of wasteful practices and would report them to Head Office. Whatever was discovered

would then be investigated and solutions or recom-
mendations would then be put forward. I think
many people would enjoy being a part of something
like that because they could make a difference. They
could help change something that could be wasteful.

It's my belief that we've all been desensitized to
some degree in regards to waste in society. We've
seen it so much all of our lives that it becomes too
easy to just ignore it or think that there's nothing we
can do about it. It might seem like just a little bit of
waste and it's not going to make any difference but if
you put all those little bits together, it makes a BIG
difference. Just about everything that we do waste
can be reused or converted into something else.

There's a part of my journey that I'm very proud
of and it has to do with waste. A number of years
ago I was grocery shopping in a major food store
when I noticed an employee in the Produce
Department had a half box of ripe bananas on his
cart. I asked what he was going to do with them and
he said, "Throw them away." Shocked, I asked if I
could buy them and he replied, "Sure. How about
50¢?" After that, I started checking out what ripe
produce I could buy cheap. I began to realize that
these stores throw away an awful lot of good food,
It's not all rotten, it's just ripe and ready to eat. I
decided to try and divert some of this food to people
who really needed it. There was a place in
Vancouver run by Nuns who fed needy people every
day and I decided to take the food there. It started
out slowly but, after a while, I was collecting quite a
bit of food. The sisters couldn't handle it all through

their kitchen so I began just stopping at the front of the mission where the people lined up for their meals. I was amazed and humbled to witness these people empty a pickup truck load of fresh produce in about five minutes. I would stand there handing out plastic shopping bags as fast as I could. Many people thanked me for what I was doing and I began to get to know some of the street people down there.

I remember one day a rather rough looking gentleman came up to me with two bags of produce and said, "Thanks man. This is the best day of my life." I realized at that moment just how much I take for granted and how lucky I really am. I took a truck load of fresh fruits and vegetables downtown once a week for a year and a half. I must say, to their credit, most of the produce managers were very cooperative. They would get their employees to save the ripe stuff for me. I always let them know what day I would be coming down. I had a route of stores that I would stop at on that scheduled day. On the best day I had, I collected 19 cases of bananas alone, 17 were from one store. With all the other food I collected on that day I had literally close to a ton of produce.

Eventually I couldn't continue because I did it totally on my own time and with my own money. Regrettably I had to stop. I also started to feel resistance from some of the stores. It seemed that higher-up management didn't like me bringing attention to the fact of how much they really did waste. That was the whole point in the beginning, to bring attention to the waste.

When I look back on that period of time, I'm

thankful that I was able to feed so many people.

I seem to keep drifting back to the subject of Balance. I think it's an important point. When things get out of balance, that's when problems are created. When you think about it, that's where just about all the world's problems stem from. Power, money, energy, pollution, population, racial and gender equality, wealth, poverty, extinctions, crime, violence, environment. The list could go on and on but I believe it all comes down to man pushing the scales too far to one side and tipping it out of balance. It's just like the "Balance of Nature". The reason it balances out is because Man isn't in the equation anymore. We've taken ourselves out of Nature and now try to assert our dominance over it.

Now you might think I'm getting philosophical and all high and mighty. You're probably right but we have to become acutely aware of the imbalances we create and try to correct them. The easiest thing to do about any problem is to deny it exists. Unfortunately when you deny a problem exists, more often than not, the worse that problem becomes. Hate, prejudice, deceit, violence, greed and almost all other negative forces breed in silence. We can't be silent. We have to become aware and speak out. We have to try to get things back into Balance. That includes each other. Another word for Balance is Equal. We are all equal to each other. If only we could learn to stop pushing each other around. We all have the same worth so why do we keep trying to dominate each other? We all have the same rights. We are all special in our own way. If we could all

just realize that we need each other we just might be
able to fix this mess we've created.

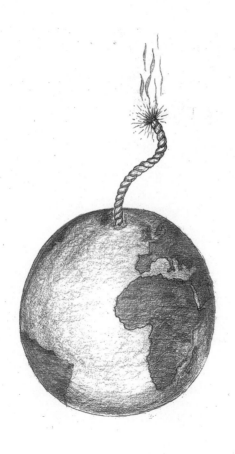

I Wish

I wish I could take every human being for a ride.
I wish I had the chance to be a planetary guide.
I wish I could take everyone no matter what their race
And stand upon the Moon and look at Earth from out in space.
Then we could see this Planet's not as big as we had thought –
That Mother Earth, our home, is truly all that we have got.
From out in space, the borders of the countries can't be seen,
The view becomes a mix of blue and brown and shades of green.
The wars and crime and violence would seem to disappear
And there would be no torture and no bloodshed and no fear.
The Earth would look so peaceful from the lunar point of view,
We'd have a chance to see the Planet Earth as something new.
We'd see her as she really is, as something to respect
And not something to dominate and poison and neglect.
I wish each person in the World could stand up there with me
And maybe then, just maybe, there's a chance we could be free.

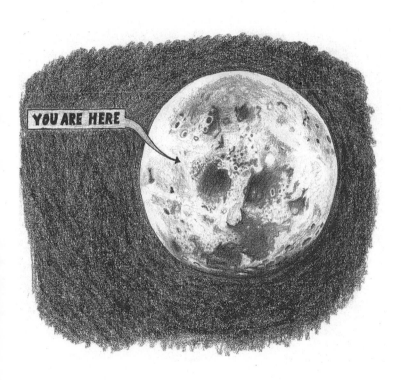

In my opinion, we don't get along very well. All through history it has been man against man, family against family, religion against religion, and country against country. When you think about all the problems on this planet, whether it's pollution, energy shortages, transportation problems, communication, food supplies, population control or clean water availability, if we could eliminate conflict we would have all the money, power and resources we would need to solve all the world's problems.

Think about it. How much money does every country in the world spend on arming itself? Millions, billions, trillions. Look at how much money went into the Nuclear Arms Race. There's probably enough nuclear warheads on this planet to destroy every living thing a thousand times over. Just a bit too much overkill, don't you think? Not to mention all the chemical weapons, biological weapons and good old-fashioned bang-bang shoot-'em-up artillery. Why do we have all this fire power? Because we don't get along very well. Why not? Because we've divided ourselves up into little groups. Each group saying "We're right and you're wrong and there's nothing you can do about it."

Well, I say "Hold it. Wait a minute." We're not Jews and Gentiles. We're not Catholics and Protestants. We're not Americans and Russians. We're not Iraquis and Kuwaities. We're not black and white. We're not us and them. We're all Earthlings. We're all Human Beings. We're all part of the Human Family.

As a matter of fact, putting the biblical Adam and Eve story aside, there was a landmark genetic study done in 1987 by scientists of the University of California at Berkley. They compared a type of DNA passed down in females that remains unchanged through generations. Women were tested from around the world and the study suggests the origin of all people can be traced back to one woman in Africa about 200,000 years ago. It's called the Eve Hypothesis. Of course, other experts challenged the theory and have their own theories but if the Eve Hypothesis is correct, then we ARE all related. We are literally ONE FAMILY.

Anyway, the point is, regardless of all the theories, we are all in this together. Either we get our act together or we're in a lot of trouble.

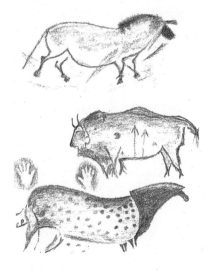

As One

The world sometimes is really not a pretty place
         to live
A lot of people only take, they never want to give
They're fighting with their fellow man, they torture,
         kill and maim
They're warring with their neighbours, they're
         killing in God's name
Why can't we see ourselves as ONE, we're all
         the same to me
We're brothers and we're sisters, we're all one
         big family
We're human beings stranded on this island
         out in space
We're all the same, no matter what our colour
         or our race
The borders of this World are what have put us
         in this spot
We can't divide up Mother Earth, it's all that
         we have got
We have to work together, try to solve our
         problems here
Destroying Planet Earth is truly now my
         biggest fear
But if we help each other and try not to kill
         and fight
Then we can turn this mess around and finally
         do what's right
Instead of dreaded enemies, then we could all
         be friends
I pray, that I will see the day, when all
         the warring ends

The Life Guy

A Journey

I mentioned at the start of this book that I've been writing a column for a 'good news' newspaper called "Know News". Nicole Whitney, the publisher of the Vancouver, BC based paper, decided to change its name in February 1999 from "Know News" to "The Phoenix" because of the somewhat negative connotation inherent in the word "Know". Whenever I told someone about the paper, I would spell out the work 'know'. K-N-O-W News not NO News.

I'm very thankful for the opportunity to be able to write about issues that are important to me and have them printed in a timely, much needed, uplifting, positive newspaper. I'm also humbled and honored to have been dubbed the "Life Guy".

At the risk of repeating myself, I've decided to reprint my columns here in this book for a couple of reasons. First, they are a continuation of my journey. They are also an extension of this book. Almost everything in this book was written before I started writing the columns. Even though I talk about issues I've already touched on, they're covered in a bit more detail or from a different perspective. I also believe they are important issues. Finally, I have to say I'm proud of them and I wanted to share them with you. I hope you enjoy them.

YOU'RE IN CHARGE

I used to think that a journey was something that you went on like a holiday. Maybe it was on a train or an airplane, on foot, perhaps horseback. A journey; a vacation; somewhere you went. It had a beginning and an end. I've come to realize that there is another much more important journey: The Journey of Life. This journey also has a beginning and an end. It's all about getting from point "A" to point "B" with point "A" being conception and point "B" being death. Many people believe our journey continues beyond the grave but I'm not really qualified to talk about the hereafter because I'm still in the here-and-now. I hope that our journey does continue for it would be nice to think that even death doesn't kill the human spirit. But for now we're here plodding along on our journey of life. The way I look at it, we're actually on two trips at the same time: the collective human journey which refers to the direction which we as a race are going together and the individual journeys of us all which head off in different directions.

Personally, my journey is usually going in different directions at the same time. I guess that's why I have trouble finishing things sometimes. I have too many things going on all at once. I guess in some ways that's good because I can never honestly say, "I'm bored". I used to think I wasn't in control of my journey. Actually I didn't know I was on one. I thought I was being catapulted here and shoved

163

there. I had given up control of my life and allowed everyone else to push me around. The key word there is *allowed*. I used to think I didn't have a choice but now I know better. No one can really tell you what to do unless you allow him or her to. We can't decide one day that we're not going to obey traffic lights or we're not going to pay taxes or abide by the laws of the land. Well, we *could* but there would be societal imposed consequences for our actions. Our culture is based on freedom but governed by rules. Since the alternative is anarchy, that's okay. So once we've given up our "required amount" of control to fit into society, we're in charge of everything else. It's true that sometimes circumstance doesn't give us the most favourable set of choices to choose from but it is still OUR choice. We are in control. I used to give up all my control, throw my hands up in the air and say, "What's the use?" I'd lose faith and hope for the future because I gave up control.

Assertiveness is something that has helped establish control in my life. I used to be too willing to "give in" on an issue and not defend my own thoughts and beliefs. I've always been somewhat passive in my demeanor and was intimidated by aggression. The trouble was confusing assertiveness with aggression. The funny thing is they are actually opposites. Aggression is offensiveness. Assertiveness is defensiveness.

Perhaps in the old days choices were simpler. We live in a complicated society and while in some ways life is very easy due to technological advancements, it can be more difficult because of it. In the past, much of our time, energy and attention were paid to the business of survival. Food, clothing and shelter were a priority. Today, most of that stuff is already taken care of. Society is moving at an accelerating speed with a unparalleled number of choices at our feet. Instead of getting overwhelmed, I get excited about having so many to pick from. When I went to school, there were no computer courses available. Now the number of career choices in that field alone is staggering. Even though I do a radio show on the Internet, I'm still fairly computer illiterate but I'm learning. I can choose to learn as much as I want or choose to learn nothing at all. I can choose to work with computers or I can become a farmer. Actually in my case, I'm trying to do both. I love gardening, need to buy a tractor and am in the process of convincing my wife that "goats are a good thing". It all comes down to my choice. No one else is in charge.

I've spent too much time letting people push my buttons, pull my strings and make choices for me. I'm the one that has to live my life. I'm the one that has to be responsible for my decisions. No one is going to live my life for me. So, in the end, I'm in control of my journey and you're in control of yours. Sometimes it may not feel that way. Someone may be trying to push your buttons or asking you to do something that you think is wrong. Someone else may want to take control of your life. Just remember one thing: *you're in charge.* It's YOUR life. It's your journey. Take the reins. Get behind the wheel. Put your foot on the gas and have a safe trip. See you on the road.

- September 1998

GRATITUDE IS A GREAT ATTITUDE

I'm a very lucky person. I'm extremely thankful for the gifts that have been given me. I'm thankful for the experiences that have been laid before me. Those experiences weren't all pleasant. As a matter of fact, some were downright horrible. I've experienced the deaths of loved ones including my son and my brother. I've felt the pain of abuse on many different levels. I've lived through drug and alcohol dependency. I know what it feels like to have a low self-esteem and low self-worth. I've seen how painful life can be. I'm very thankful for that. Now, that may sound strange being thankful for the pain throughout my life but if I had not been through the pain, I don't think I could truly appreciate the joy. By seeing the ugliness of life, it helped me to appreciate the beauty. The death of my son has helped me to realize how precious life really is.

All the events and experiences in my life have helped shape my outlook and attitude. I wouldn't want to change that. I've said many times that I wouldn't want to relive all those painful experiences but if I had a magic wand and could change my past, I wouldn't change a thing. All those painful events have contributed to who I am today. The attitude I have towards myself is quite different today than in the past. I like myself today. I'm proud of who I am and what I do. I stand up for myself and assert my right to be respected. I like my life. No. Wait. I LOVE my life. Sometimes I have to stop and take a look at how my life is going in comparison to how it used to be. It amazes me how things have changed. I haven't really changed physically but the way my mind sees life in general has changed dramatically. The most important change has been in how I view myself. In the past I didn't really like who I was. Everybody else seemed to like Randy but *Randy didn't like himself.*

I was always overly concerned about what people thought of me. I would be careful to say the right thing so I could fit in and be accepted. The trouble was, I didn't accept myself. When you're stumbling through life with a low self-esteem it becomes very hard to get anywhere. Happiness and contentment seem out of the question. Daily living becomes a major struggle.

Fortunately, through a long chain of events, I was able to get a grasp on a healthier way of looking at life. I stopped beating myself up for making mistakes. I began to realize that it's not what someone else thinks about me that's important: it's what I think about myself that counts. I started to see that no one was going to come along and live my life for me. I had to take control, make my own decisions, take actions based upon those decisions and then take responsibility for my actions. Responsibility was always something I had difficulty with. Nobody said life was going to be easy.

Actually, that's what makes life interesting. It would be pretty boring if everything was easy. Have you ever noticed that when something is just given to you, it doesn't seem to have as much value compared to something that you struggled and worked hard for? When something is difficult to achieve, it is usually appreciated more.

I'm thankful that the reality of life gave me a good shaking. I'm grateful that I was given a big wake up call. It's as if somebody upstairs was saying, "Excuse me! You better get your act together! Life is short. Use it while you've got a chance."

There have been times in my life that have been very difficult. I'm grateful for the ups and downs, pain and joys, tears and laughter, and sometimes chaos of everyday life. I guess, in the end, it all comes down to your attitude towards life. Generally speaking, my life is GREAT but, there are times it really sucks. Life is like a roller coaster. You have your ups and downs. So when you're at the bottom of the hill, instead of being bummed out about it, just remember its part of the ride. Life is supposed to be like that. It wouldn't be very much fun if it was all too easy now would it?

See you on the roller coaster.

- October 1998

THE MANY FACETS OF INTEGRITY

The dictionary defines integrity as: 1). Honesty or sincerity; uprightness; 2). Undivided or unbroken condition; completeness; wholeness; entirety. Even though the second definition refers to integrity in terms of an object or thing as in the integrity of a piece of art or manuscript, I believe it perfectly states how we come into this world. As newborns we are whole, complete and more importantly, unbroken. We are pure. We are honest. When we are hungry or wet we cry. When we are happy we smile. We don't manipulate or lie. We don't cheat. We don't hurt others on purpose.

So what happens? Why do we lose that? I suppose there are a lot of reasons; the need to survive, competition, one-upmanship and of course, the way we're treated by fellow human beings. I think one of the biggest factors is competition. As babies grow into toddlers they become more possessive of their belongings. Who hasn't heard a two year old with a toy loudly proclaim "Mine, mine!" Early on we learn to defend ourselves and to protect what we see as ours – not just in a material sense, but our relationships with family and friends, jobs and everything else seems to need to be protected in some way. We are afraid that someone may come along and take what we see as ours.

The problem is when people become greedy and want more. They never seem to be satisfied. Not that wanting more is a bad thing but sometimes people make it the most important thing. No matter how much power, possessions or money some people have, they still want more. Have you ever heard of the billionaire who phoned all his factories and told them to stop making a profit because he had enough money? No? Neither have I. I have heard of businesses that weren't making enough profit so they cut back on staff. They don't call that "laying off". They call it "downsizing". It looks bad in the quarterly report if they say "Our profits are up but we had to throw 200 people out in the street". The HUMAN element is most often taken out to make it more palatable. "Laying off" is people. "Downsizing" is the company.

Then there is integrity in government. Wow, there's an oxymoron. If companies ran their businesses like most governments do, they would be out of business. Let's face it. Government is business. They consistently run deficits, overspend, give golden handshakes to the faithful, make up their own rules and generally do a poor job of being fair and equitable. Most people have the impression that once someone becomes elected, whatever morals they had go out the window and from that moment on, they tow the party line. To some extent that may be true. Not to say all politicians lack integrity, some are fighting for what they believe in and genuinely work for the good of the people. Yet some politicians are, shall we say, less than credible. Then there is integrity (or lack there-of) in the justice system: the lawyers, police, judges and criminals. This is a story unto itself.

How about integrity in the media? In the pursuit of a juicy story some media sources have chosen to pursue stories for entertainment purposes rather than newsworthy information. The negative sensationalism of the news has seriously undermined the credibility of the media as a whole, which is one of the reasons Darryl and I have put together our Erthtones (Internet) radio show. With a potential audience of people from all around the world, we hope in some small way to help the integrity of human beings as well as that of the media. We only promote positive news and thoughts. Nobody gets shot or dies on our show. Nobody commits armed robbery, adultery or perjury. We are a negativity-free radio program. This paper is a negativity-free-zone and I'm proud to be a contributing party.

Personal integrity is something most people don't give much thought to. What does personal integrity mean to you? What does it mean to me? I think personal integrity means doing the RIGHT thing. If a cashier gives me too much change, I tell that person. I hold doors open for strangers. If something looks unsafe, I bring it to someone's attention. If I find a lost item, I try to find the owner. I try to be respectful of others. I try to be honest at all times. I try to be fair. Notice I said *try*. I'm not perfect. I still make mistakes. Sometimes it's hard to tell the truth about everything. Sometimes the truth hurts people's feelings. I try not to hurt other people. In short, I try to treat people the way I want them to treat me. I always try to maintain my own personal integrity. I try my best to do the RIGHT thing. To me, that is integrity!

- *November 1998*

GIVING IS WHAT IT TAKES

Have you ever heard of someone described as being a very "giving person"? Does that mean they're always giving away their stuff or they're handing out presents all the time? No, I don't think so. They may give someone a gift once in a while but I think the term "giving person" doesn't have anything to do with material goods at all. I believe it refers to the best kind of giving – giving of yourself. That to me is the highest form of giving. Taking the time in this hectic world to help out your fellow human being. It could be something simple like taking the time to listen to someone who really needs to talk. Maybe it's a child, teenager, coworker or an elder. It could be anybody. Many people in this world are frustrated, annoyed, disillusioned or depressed because they feel no one is listening to them. A lot of people don't want to hear what you have to say. They engage in conversation just so they can voice their own views and opinions. While you're talking, they're waiting for you to take a breath so they can jump in and interrupt. They're not really listening. It's too bad because they're probably talking to someone who just wants to be heard.

I volunteered over 300 hours answering calls at the Langley Crisis Line. I used to think, probably like most other people, that a Crisis Line was for emergencies only. I was under the impression that you had to be on the verge of suicide before you could call. After I went through the training and spent some time on the phones, I realized the main function of a Crisis Line is to listen, to hear what the person is saying and use empathy. What the person phoning probably needs most is for someone to understand what they are going through and to empathize with their situation. It was amazing the wide diversity of calls that came through but they almost all boiled down to being a person who needed someone to listen to them. I believe that listening doesn't come naturally for most people. Just ask any parent. They've probably said things like "You're not listening to me. When I'm talking to you, I expect you to listen." Do we really listen to each other though? Do we really hear and understand what the other person is saying? Something I've said to my son is "If you're talking, you're not listening. If you're not listening, you're not learning." Listening is learning. When you listen, both parties benefit. One person is being heard and understood. The other person is learning something from the exchange. Wow! Wouldn't it be a wonderful world if all conversations went like that? Listening is "giving" someone your attention.

Another way of "giving" of yourself is volunteering. I believe that volunteers are the largest group of unsung heroes we have in society. I don't know the exact figure but there are thousands if not millions of hours donated every year by volunteers across the country. To me, volunteering embodies the essence of "giving". Helping each other without expecting anything in return. Then again, volunteers do benefit. Giving your time and energy to a cause that you believe in can be a very rewarding experience. I, for one, would like to say to all volunteers around the world, "Thank you. I salute you. Keep up the good work."

There are lots of ways to be giving of yourself. Help a friend move, be a mentor for someone, coach a sports team, be a big brother or sister, call a friend or your parents for no reason except just to say hi and to see how they're doing. Or even wait that extra four seconds to hold the door for someone behind you. One of the best ways to give of yourself is to take the time to make someone a gift. Seeing as this is the "Season of Giving", instead of buying all your Christmas gifts, try making some. I think that when someone takes the time and energy to create a special gift with their own two hands, it has much more meaning. They have put some of themselves into that gift. Whatever you do be it bake, carve, draw, write, color, arts and crafts, macramé, knit, sew...Just do it!! I'm sure it will be appreciated. That includes homemade cards as well. Hallmark won't go out of business if I say this but instead of trying to find a card that says something close to what you want to say, take the time to make a card and write exactly what you want to say.

Remember, giving is not necessarily material goods, it sometimes is just a kind word or thought. My Christmas gift to you is only words but they do come from the heart. "Take care of yourself, have a safe and happy holiday and give a part of yourself to someone this season."

- December 1998

A CHANGE FOR THE BETTER

When you think of January and the New Year you often think of New Year's Resolutions. People get caught up in the tradition of New Year's Resolutions and start saying things like "This year I'm going to quit smoking and lose some weight. I'm going to stop biting my nails. I'm going to cut down on my fat intake. This year I'm going to start exercising regularly." If you notice, all those things are positive improvements. I've never heard anyone make a New Year's Resolution like "This year I'm just going to let myself go. I'm going to lose my job and alienate all my friends." It seems to me, a resolution is about improving yourself in some way. If you break up the word resolution to re-solution, it then means trying again to solve a problem. If you make a resolution, you already know what the problem is; you're just trying to solve it. If so many people already know what the problem is, why are New Year's Resolutions so hard to keep?

Sometimes people even make jokes about resolutions because they know they won't stick to them. An example would be "My New Year's Resolution this year is to stop making New Year's Resolutions." Why is that? Why do a lot of people have trouble making lasting positive improvements in themselves? I suppose there are many answers to that question and one is "It's easier to just keep doing what you've always done even if it's unsafe or unhealthy." It sounds silly even saying that but it's true. Change isn't always easy. To change something about your-self would mean being uncomfortable for a while. It means doing things you've never done before which brings in fear of the unknown. People are creatures of habit and change involves not know what is going to happen to them. People don't like not knowing. Not knowing implies risk. Risk means potential loss. I don't think anybody enjoys losing so to avoid it, they don't risk. If there is no risk, there is no change. If there is no change, then the problem is left unre-solved. If left unattended, problems have a way of solving themselves. The problem with that is the con-sequence of an ignored problem is usually not the most desirable outcome. The status quo is often easi-er in the short term but an unattended problem can get way out of hand. I guess a good analogy would be cancer. Nobody wants to have it happen to them. It would be easier to not check for the signs and hope it doesn't happen to you. If it does, however, and you've ignored the signs, it may be too late. The con-sequences of that could be death – not a desirable outcome. As a matter of fact there are a couple of types of cancer that run in my family. Of course I hope it doesn't happen to me and the check-ups for these cancers are not exactly pleasant but if I ignore it, I could pay with my life. So what are my choices? Be uncomfortable during the check-ups and possibly live a lot longer or ignore the possibility of it hap-pening to me and potentially die sooner. I'll let you guess which choice I went with.

Most of the time, change is a choice. You can choose to go with change or choose to go against it.

People are often resistant to change but without it, we would be doomed. Change is everything. It's inevitable. Nothing stays the same. Everything is constantly changing. One of the factors that has made the human race so successful is humans have the ability to adapt to change. It may not always be easy but change is necessary for progress. Improvement comes from change.

When I look back on my life, it amazes me how much I've changed. Physically I'm not all that different but the way I look at the world has changed dramatically. I guess the way I look at myself has changed the most. For a large part of my life, I didn't like who I was and I didn't accept myself. It took a while but the journey I've been on has allowed me to see that I'm just a human being like everybody else. I make mistakes. I learn. I laugh. I cry. I'm glad that I took risks. I allowed myself to be vulnerable. I stepped outside my "comfort zone" and let myself adapt to changes I was going through. It certainly wasn't easy but I'm thankful for those changes. They helped make me a better person. They helped me be more comfortable with who I am.

If changing old habits is difficult for you, I would think that means you're normal. Just go easy on yourself. Don't set yourself up to fail. Don't attempt to change too much too quickly. Allow yourself time to adjust and adapt. If you want to make a New Year's Resolution, pick something do-able. Choose something you really want to change and stick to it. Change is certainly possible but make sure you pick something you actually have control over. Obviously some things are beyond our control. It's not a good idea to make a resolution like "This year I'm going to make myself taller." If something is bothering you, really look at it and think about what it is that you want to change. Ask yourself questions like "What don't I like about this? What can I do to change it? Do I really want to change it? What steps do I have to take? What do I do first? If I can't change it, what other options do I have?"

If I were going to make a resolution this year, it wouldn't be something I want to change. It would be something I want to continue. My resolution would be "This year I will continue to freely embrace the changes in my life." After all, there's always room for improvement, right?

- *January 1999*

WHAT IS LOVE?

When I found out that "LOVE" would be this month's theme, I thought, "Well, that should be easy to write about. Love is all around us." Love is the number one song lyric subject as in "Love is in the Air", "All You Need is Love", "Everybody Loves Somebody Sometime", "Love is the Drug", "To Sir, With Love", "I Love You", he loves her, you love me, she loves him, yada, yada, yada. So if more songs have been written about love than anything else, writing a column about it shouldn't be that hard, right?

Then I really started thinking about love. What is it about love that is so powerful? What IS love? If you want information, where do you go these days? The Internet, of course. So off to my computer I go and type in the words "What is love?" As I scanned down the list and sampled some of the sites it seemed to me that these other people didn't really know what love is either. They knew what love DID. They knew what it FELT like. They knew what it made them DO. They knew a lot ABOUT love. But what IS it? Why is it? Why is it that we feel love? Do animals feel love? I don't think so. It doesn't seem like they do. In the animal world, for the most part, males are genetic dispensers. Any male/female bonding usually involves reproduction. If there is love in the animal world, it is probably between mother and baby. Then again, that nurturing could be considered instinct. I don't know if animals feel love but I know that

humans do. Why? Go with me for a minute on this –
I think it has something to do with the length of time
it takes to raise a human child. Love is the emotional
bond that holds two people together long enough to
reproduce and nurture an offspring. It's the emotional glue that keeps the species going. Or is that lust?
Wait. That's a whole other column. I think in the
original scope of things, love was meant to be procre-
ation cement. Not very romantic, is it?

When writers don't know something, they usually just make it up. I don't know where love came
from so I made up my own little legend entitled
"How Humans Got Love". It goes like this:

One day, God was sitting around after the big
"Creation" thing looking at all His beautiful work.
He could see that these humans were a lot more
complicated than He first thought. He realized it
would take two parents to raise a healthy child to the
point of adulthood. He needed to give them something special so He created the most beautiful feeling
in the world. He called it Love. He gave it to the
humans so the adults would have a wonderful lasting bond to share and keep them together. The feeling of love was so beautiful and powerful, it spread
to all human relationships. Soon, every human
being had the ability to love someone. The End.

That's my story and I'm stickin' to it. (Hey,
another song title.)

When you think about it, raising a child through
to the level of independence is a HUGE investment in
terms of time and energy (not to mention$$). There
needed to be some kind of emotional payback to
maintain the output of energy required. We spend

more time raising our young than any other organism on this planet.

When I think about love, I usually think about the man/woman love first. Obviously there are many types of love. I love my wife. I love my children. I love my mom. I love my father even though he has passed away. I love my brother – he's gone too. I love my job. I love gardening. Hey, I even love my mother-in-law.☺ It's fairly clear that all those relationships are very different. We still apply the word love to them. I guess that's what love really is: A relationship. I believe that love is supposed to be a healthy respectful heartfelt relationship but sometimes "Love Hurts", "Love Stinks", and love sometimes sucks. Sometimes you love someone who can't/won't/doesn't love you back. But, I feel that love is a deep subconscious connection that we have with another person or thing.

Something else that people love is their animals. There are cat lovers, dog lovers, horse lovers, bird lovers. People seem to bond with animals. They LOVE their animals.

There is yet another kind of love that most people never talk or even think about. I'm sure some people have never even felt it. That love is self-love. I'm not referring to an overblown, self-absorbed, conceited ego. I simply mean loving and accepting yourself. I know for most of my life, loving and accepting myself was not my reality. I was more into self-hate than self-love. Funny thing was, everybody else seemed to like me. I just didn't like myself. The reasons for my lack of self-love and acceptance were mostly due to the experiences I had been through in my life and my reluctance to let go of the past. I was constantly beating myself up for mistakes I had made. It's pretty hard to love and accept yourself when you're always thinking, "What a failure I am", "What a jerk I've been", "How could I have been so stupid?", "What's the matter with me?" All that does is bring in self-doubt, self-blame and self-ridicule. A far cry from the goal of self-love. We make mistakes. That's what humans do. Actually many products, inventions and theories came from a direct result of mistakes. Mistakes teach us what to do what not to do. An aid to achieving self-love is accepting that you're just a human being. You're going to make mistakes. That's okay. Don't beat yourself up. You deserve respect. You deserve to be treated fairly. You deserve to be loved – especially by yourself.

As the old saying goes, "The only person you're always going to have in your life is you." Everybody else can come and go but YOU will always be there. You can spend the rest of your life with someone you dislike or someone that you love. In order for you to have a healthy respectful long-term relationship between yourself and anyone else, self-love is critical. It is one of the most important contributions you can make to the nourishment of a lasting relationship with another person.

It's not always easy to love yourself but it's worth it. Just "Put a Little Love in Your Heart". Tap into the "Power of Love". I think Stephen Stills said it best – "if you can't be with the one you love, honey, 'Love the One You're With'." (Pssst!! That would be YOU.)

- *February 1999*

Conclusion

A Journey

S o what does all this mean? What am I trying to say to you? What is the key to a better life? What IS the answer? Well, I think the fundamental problem with trying to find the answer to the proverbial question "What is the meaning of life?" is that the answer is different for everyone. What works for me may not work for you. What I find exciting and stimulating, you may find totally boring. What feels good for me might feel bad for you and vice versa. The problem is we all look at things differently. We see with our eyes but we interpret what we see through our past memories and experiences. What I see as beautiful, you may see as ugly.

Unfortunately, for the Human Race, that's good and bad at the same time. It's good because we act independently. We have our own thoughts and ideas. Out of those ideas come concepts, theories, inventions and products. Seeing the world differently and acting independently stimulates our imaginations and creative processes.

The bad side to all of this is we act independently. We don't always want to work together. We create divisions and walls around ourselves. We like to have our own space as groups and as individuals. We seem to have a desire to stand alone – to make it all by ourselves – to prove that we can do it without anyone's help or input. To show that we have the ability to take care of ourselves. The problem is we can't do everything all by ourselves. We need each other. We are social beings. We work best by working together, helping each other and sharing our experiences. That is what has made the Human Race so successful. Cooperation.

Now, obviously if you look at human history, we haven't always cooperated with each other. Imagine if we had. Think for a moment at what we could have accomplished by now if we hadn't spent all that time and energy fighting and killing each other.

I like to watch documentaries about human history, anthropology and cultural diversity. Human history is MY history. I am a member of the Human Race and so are you. I know that working together WE can accomplish anything we put our collective minds to.

Physics states that each action has an equal and opposite reaction. I believe that in human behaviour each action has a consequence. Good and bad. I think a lot of people believe that their actions don't matter. Somehow what they say or do doesn't count or mean anything. I believe that every little action does count. It DOES matter what people say and do because everyone is involved and connected in a continuous chain of actions and consequences that becomes human history. You DO count. You DO matter. What you say and do truly is important to all of us. You are a part of human history.

This book isn't really about what the Human Race can do. It's more about what each of us can do individually. Obviously this book contains my words and thoughts about my experiences. However, I didn't put these words down on paper just so I could tell you about my life or share my poetry with you. What I hoped to do was to help make someone's life just a little bit easier. What I wanted to show was although things may seem overwhelming and insurmountable, they don't always have to stay that way. What I hoped to illustrate was that life CAN get better if you make the right choices.

Even though I believe that a force greater than myself is overseeing my life, I still believe that I am ultimately responsible for my life's outcome. If I hadn't made the choices about changing my lifestyle and behaviour back then, I could very well have ended up like my brother, Lloyd – dead at an early age. I realize that my actions directly affect the outcome of my destiny. I know now that I am truly in control of my life or should I say I am in control of my choices. Sometimes events come into my life that I have no control over. I do, however, have control over the choices I make regarding those events and how I deal with them. It can be all too easy to be overwhelmed by a situation and give up or run away from it without really thinking about what the best course of action would be. Sometimes running away is the best thing to do but not very often. It's usually best to face something, objectively look at it and make a responsible informed decision. That may sound great in theory but it's not always easy to deal with an uncomfortable situation and remain objective. Sometimes it's easier to keep yourself ignorant of the facts. As the old saying goes "Ignorance is bliss". Ignorance isn't bliss. Ignorance means not having the tools at your disposal to help resolve problems that are having an affect on your life. Ignorance means being unaware. The trick is to gain the knowledge you need to help alleviate the stress and/or crisis. The sources of stress in our lives are wide and varied. Most can be addressed by first understanding what they are and then doing something about it. It's the "doing something about it" that's the hard part. Changing our thought patterns and habits can be difficult. It's not easy to change the way we react to certain stimuli or situations but the payoff can be worth it. By using empathy and by looking at something from another person's point of view, even just briefly, can bring you better understanding and insight about a situation. By understanding something better, you're more likely to be less stressed out by it. Stress can cloud our reasoning ability and make us react in ways we normally wouldn't. We have to take responsibility for our own actions.

Problems don't usually resolve themselves. Throughout history there have been problems. Problems will continue. Maybe instead of calling them problems, we should refer to them as "situations that require attention." That's really what they are. If someone has a drug problem, it doesn't have to be permanent. If someone has a drinking problem, it can be addressed. If someone has a behavioural problem, appropriate measures can be taken. Problems are situations that require attention. The problem with most problems is that they don't get enough attention or the right kind of attention. Every situation is different. The measures taken need to be tailored to that particular situation. You wouldn't send a guy with a broken leg to see a psychologist. His problem isn't in his mind. His leg is broken.

I believe that many people who have problems or "situations that require attention," know what those problems are and know what they need to do about them. For one reason or another, they find it difficult to take the necessary steps to address the situation. I believe that most people know what they NEED. The trouble is, they are usually controlled by what they WANT. It seems a lot of people confuse Needs with Wants. Needs keep us alive. Wants are everything else.

What about me? What do I want? I want to see the world become a better place to live in. I want to remain proud of myself for making healthy choices. I want to see my children grow up with healthy minds and bodies. I want to continue being creative in different areas of my life. I want to truly enjoy my life. I want to help one human being on their journey of life be more comfortable and happy.

What about you? What do you want?

Good luck on your journey,

Randy Thompson

Poetry Index